CLINICAL BIOSTATISTICS
and epidemiology
MADE RIDICULOUSLY SIMPLE

Ann Weaver, PhD
Professor, Statistics and Research
Program Chair of Research and Statistics
Argosy University, Sarasota FL

Stephen Goldberg, MD
Professor Emeritus
University of Miami
Miller School of Medicine
Miami FL

MEDMASTER

Made in the United States of America

Published by
MedMaster, Inc.
3389 Sheridan Street, #243
Hollywood, FL 33021

ISBN: 978-1-962445-33-7
eISBN: 978-1-962445-34-4

Cover design: Jordan Collver and Owen Watts
Proofreading: Phyllis Goldenberg

To JERRY and to JOHN

CONTENTS

PREFACE

This book is a brief, intuitive approach to clinical biostatistics, not just to pass the medical Boards, but also to improve patient care by assisting practitioners in evaluating medical literature.

Drug representatives continually approach medical practitioners with biased views; side effects are often minimized and benefits are exaggerated. Patients request drugs advocated on TV; research studies contradict one another. Is one drug really better than another? Is the new drug worth the extra expense? Does the drug or procedure cause more harm than good? There's a lot of bad information out there.

Physicians and other health care practitioners should not only understand a research paper's Abstract and Conclusions sections, but also the Materials and Methods section. This requires understanding of key biostatistics concepts and the pitfalls of biostatistics. Reviewers of research articles may be experts in the field of study, but are not necessarily experts in biostatistics; a poor paper frequently gets through reviewer scrutiny.

Learning a lot of math can be time-consuming and the medical practitioner generally does not have the time for this. Fortunately, there is not much math that the medical practitioner needs to know. The intuitive concepts are the most important and the easiest to learn and retain. This book minimizes math and emphasizes concepts.

In evaluating research, the practitioner needs to ask these four questions:

1. Is this the best research design (prospective, retrospective study, etc.), considering the aims of the study?
2. Is this the best statistical test to analyze the data (t-test, ANOVA, etc.)?
3. What do the results mean (mean, median, mode, standard deviation, SEM, confidence limits, p-values, F statistic, chi-square, etc.)?
4. Are the researchers' conclusions correct?

PART I
INTRODUCTION

CHAPTER 1. TERMINOLOGY

Population, Sample, and Element

A **population** is an entire group of people or data you want to understand. The population of diabetics in the USA is quite large; the population of people in the world with smallpox is quite small.

A **sample** is a subgroup of the whole (e.g. all diabetics in a single town, as opposed to the country). An **element** (or a **case** or **data point**) is a single observation (e.g. a single patient with diabetes).

Descriptive vs. Inferential Statistics

Descriptive statistics simply *describe* the data pertaining to a population or a sample, specifically the center of the data (e.g. mean, median, and mode), spread (variability of the data points), and shape of the plotted graph (e.g. symmetrical or not).

Inferential statistics tries to *infer* the features of a population from the limited data found in a sample. For instance, if you don't know the heights of 14-year-old males in the population, what can you infer from a sample of 14-year-old males about the likely average height in the population as a whole? Most of the time, we don't have good data about an entire population. It would be too time-consuming and expensive traveling throughout the United States measuring the heights of all 14-year-old males; we have to work with a sample and infer, from this limited data, the likely average height of the population. Most research is like that; the researcher does not have access to the entire population of people (or items) and has to infer from the sample to the population.

Parameter vs. Statistic

A **parameter** is a number that describes a ***P****opulation* characteristic (both words start with "**P**"), particularly its mean and standard deviation (a measure of data spread, described later). A **statistic** is a number that describes a ***S****ample* characteristic (both words start with "**S**"), such as the sample's mean and standard deviation.

In general, population values are indicated by Greek letters, while sample values are indicated by Roman letters. For instance:

μ: Population mean	M or $\overline{X}$: Sample mean
σ: Population standard deviation	SD: Sample standard deviation

Sampling Error vs. Selection Bias

Sampling error (unbiased): Even when a sample is randomly chosen from the population in an unbiased way, there is always going to be some natural variability that does not precisely reflect the population average. The heights, for instance, of all 14-year-olds are going to vary, based on heredity and environmental factors, and sometimes measuring error. Taking the average height of a small sample of 14-year-olds would not be expected to be exactly the average height of the population as a whole. This **sampling error** does not necessarily mean that a mistake has been made in the sampling process, or that it was sloppy in some way; it is only an acknowledgement that people and measurements normally vary. In medicine, most variation is due to biological variation rather than to imprecise measurements. The way to reduce sampling error is to increase the size of the sample.

Selection Bias: In *selection bias*, the researcher has not selected the sample randomly, but with a bias toward particular characteristics. For instance, S.G.'s wife often awakens with headaches in the middle of the night, but is otherwise fine. Searching one of the computer diagnostic programs for the differential diagnosis of "headaches awakening a person in the night" returns the leading diagnosis of "massive intracranial hemorrhage." Why? It is because the information in the program comes from in-hospital admissions, not from outpatient visits to the primary care physician. In-hospital admissions for headache are likely to be much more serious than headaches in patients who are not admitted to the hospital. The sampling in the computer diagnostic program was biased in favor of the more serious diagnosis, related to in-hospital admissions. With a biased selection, the conclusions about the general population will be wrong. Increasing the sample size does not correct for selection bias. You just have to be careful to avoid bias in the selection process.

Volunteers are not a random sample. They may, for instance, have particularly bad symptoms, which induced them, rather than less affected individuals, to join the study; they may be more likely to take risks. Surveys that invite people to call or write in with their opinions are likely to be biased.

Imprecision vs. Bias (Inaccuracy)

Consider the target in **Fig. 1–1**:

In A, Robin Hood's arrows have landed with great precision, clustering together. Unfortunately, the arrows are all way off the mark, striking a cow instead of the target. The arrows are *precise but biased*.

In B, the arrows are all equidistant but far away from the center of the target. The arrows are very *imprecise, but unbiased* in the sense that the average distance from the center of the target is right on the mark.

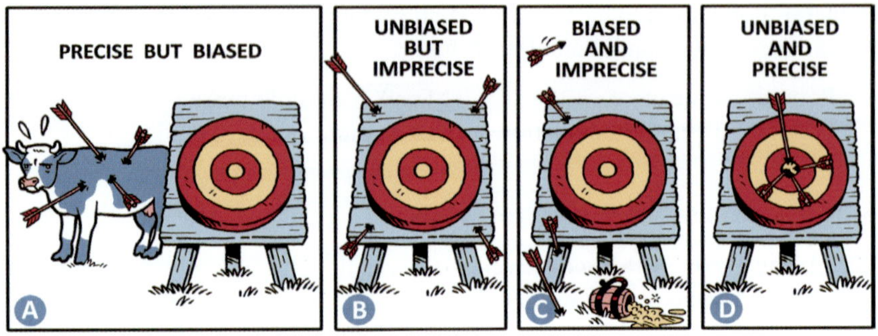

Figure 1–1. Precision and bias.

In C, after downing 6 beers, Robin's aim is both *imprecise and biased*. The arrows strike all over the place to the left of the target.

In D, the arrows are both *precise and unbiased*, being clustered together and on the mark.

Data can be that way, too. An *unbiased but imprecise* sample is one where the researcher did select a representative random sample of the population (unbiased), but there is a lot of natural variation within the sample (imprecise); there was *sampling error*. Increasing the sample size will help us know the true population average. A *precise but biased* sample is one in which the sample has little variation, but does not represent the population; there was *selection bias*. Increasing the sample size won't help selection bias.

Validity vs. Reliability

Validity, in laboratory testing, is the *accuracy* of a test. If your old blood pressure cuff repeatedly shows a reading of about 200/140 in a patient, but the actual blood pressure, using newer, modern cuffs, is 140/90, then your reading is **invalid** (inaccurate). Another way to think about it is that a *valid* instrument or test is the *right* instrument or test for the job (***mnemonic***: "valid" and "right" both have five letters).

Reliability is how *repeatable* the test is. You may have a highly accurate blood pressure cuff, but if the patient's blood pressure is highly variable, and the test needs to be repeated several times in the same visit to get a good idea of the patient's BP, then a single BP reading is an *unreliable* index of the patient's blood pressure in general. Variability in blood pressure occurs in "white-coat" hypertension, where blood pressure may vary in a clinical setting, depending on patient anxiety, which raises blood pressure.

Independent vs. Dependent Variables

A **variable** is anything that changes. An **independent variable (IV)** is one that influences the variation. A **dependent variable (DV)** is the result of applying the independent variable. For instance, when testing dosages of a drug on a patient's blood pressure, the drug dose is the independent variable; the resulting blood pressure

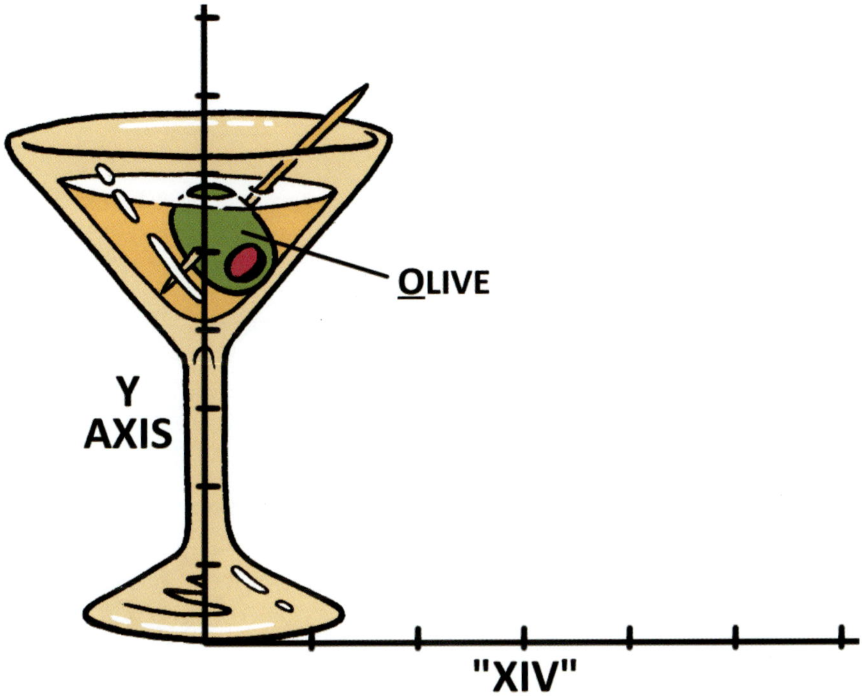

Figure 1–2. Graph axes. XIV is a mnemonic for remembering that the X axis (abscissa) generally contains the Independent Variable. The vertical stem of the martini glass is the Y axis (ordinate); the "O" in "olive" refers to "ordinate."

change is the dependent variable, which "depends" on the particular dosage. Typically, independent variables are plotted on the horizontal x axis (*abscissa*) of graphs, while dependent variables are plotted on the vertical y axis (*ordinate*).

Mnemonic: Remember the Roman numeral XIV (**Fig. 1–2**). X = x axis; IV = independent variable, which is generally placed on the x axis. Also, "**IV**" and "**I**nfluence" start with the letter "**I**" (the independent variable is the "Influence"). "**D**V," "**D**epends on," and "**D**ata" begin with the letter "**D**" (the dependent variable "Depends on" the independent variable and constitutes the "Data").

Normal (Gaussian), Skewed, and Kurtotic Curves

A "**normal**" (**Gaussian**) curve is one that has a classic bell shape (**Fig. 1–3**). Many natural phenomena have this distribution. Genetic and environmental variations, as well as errors in measurement, insure that measurements on individuals in a group are not identical, but commonly vary in a Gaussian pattern, whether in height, weight, responses to drugs, or numerous other qualities. In practice, these variations are seldom perfectly Gaussian, but if they are close enough, particularly if the sample size is large enough, you can apply many useful statistical tests on

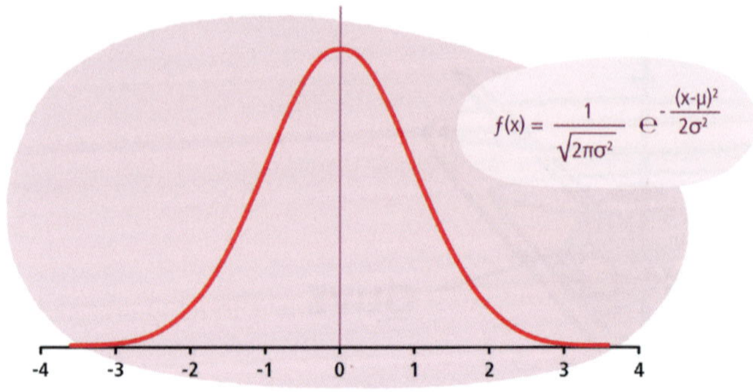

Figure 1–3. The Gaussian curve. Take a look at the mathematical formula for the curve, since you won't see it again in this book.

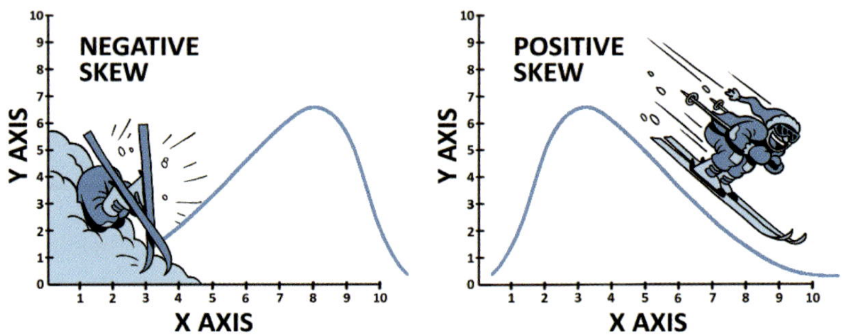

Figure 1–4. Skew. The skier positively has fun on a slope with positive skew. The experience is negative on a slope with negative skew, since the skier slams into the Y-axis. Positive skew is also called "skew to the right," since the tail extends out to the right. Similarly, negative skew is called "skew to the left."

the data. Statistical tests on data that follow a Gaussian distribution are termed **parametric** tests. When the data are not Gaussian, other kinds of tests, termed **nonparametric** tests, are used.

A curve that is not Gaussian (normal) may be **skewed** toward one side or **kurtotic** (excessively peaked or flat) (**Figs. 1–4 and 1–5**). A skew may be positive or negative (**Fig. 1–4**). **Leptokurtic** curves are excessively peaked (like the letter "l"; **positive kurtosis**), because data are more heavily concentrated around the mean than in a normal distribution. **Platykurtic** curves ("plat" rhymes with "flat") are excessively flat (**negative kurtosis**), because data are spread out and less concentrated around the mean than in a normal distribution. **(Fig. 1–5**). A curve with no excessive kurtosis, such as a Gaussian (normal) curve, is **mesokurtic**.

Sometimes a curve may be much different from a Gaussian curve, having a "**J**," "**S**" or other shape (**Fig. 1–6**). Without getting into the math, normal (Gaussian) curves have a skew of 0 and a kurtosis of 0. In general, if a curve has a skew within ± 2.0 and a kurtosis of ± 2.0, it is considered close enough to normal to be able to use parametric tests.

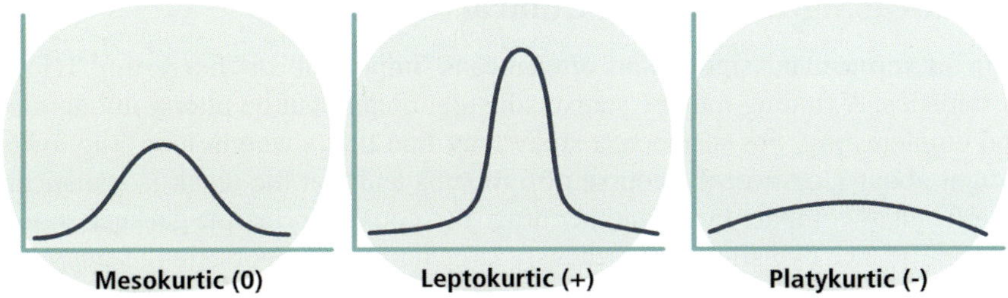

Figure 1–5. Mesokurtic (normal), leptokurtic (thin; positive kurtosis) and platykurtic (flat; negative kurtosis) curves.

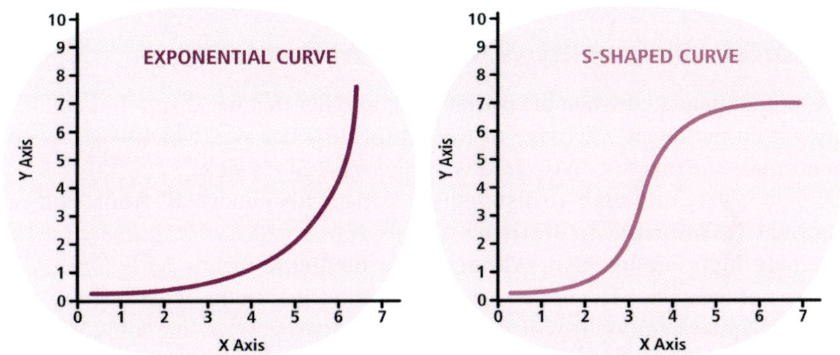

Figure 1–6. Exponential and S-shaped curves.

Multiplication and Addition Rules of Probability

Multiplication rule: What is the probability of a patient having both disease A ***and*** disease B? It is (the probability of having A) × (the probability of having B). This is the multiplication rule. For instance, if the probability of having disease A is 1 in 4 (.25; 25%) and the probability of having disease B is 1 in 3 (.33; 33%) then the probability of having *both* is .25 × .33 = .0825 (8.25%) (This assumes that A and B are independent of one another. For instance, the probability of having arteriosclerosis when you have diabetes is very high, because the two diseases are dependent, the degree of arteriosclerosis correlating with the degree of diabetic control.)

Addition rule: What is the probability of a patient having either disease A ***or*** disease B? It is (the probability of having A) + (the probability of having B), assuming the two conditions are mutually exclusive (both cannot occur at the same time). For instance, if the probability of having hypotension is .25 and the probability of hypertension is .33, then the probability of having *either* condition A or B is .25 + .33 = .58 (58%).

Note that the multiplication rule applies in an A ***and*** B situation, whereas the addition rule applies in an A ***or*** B situation.

Statistical Significance vs. Clinical Significance

In the vernacular, "significant" often means "important" or "interesting." Not so in statistics. A finding may be statistically significant, but be utterly unimportant and uninteresting. For instance, a study may find that a weight loss drug lowers weight about 1 oz over the course of 6 months and that the result is statistically significant as compared with another drug. You could in principle get such statistical significance by using an enormously large number of people in the study (one of the pitfalls in using sample sizes that are too *large*). But that degree of weight loss would hardly be important or of interest. To avoid confusion in terminology, it is better to use the term **statistically significant** rather than just "significant."

What the physician often wants to know is not whether the result is statistically significant, but whether it is **clinically significant**. That requires clinical judgment.

Statistical Abnormality vs. Clinical Abnormality

A mother panicked when the pediatrician told her that her 2 year-old child falls only within the lower 2% range of weight for girls her age, which is statistically not normal. She emotes, "My child is *not normal!* She's sick!"

Here it is very important to distinguish "statistically abnormal" from "clinically abnormal." **Abnormal in statistics** simply refers to *what is unlikely* (such as extremely high intelligence). **Abnormal in medicine** means *pathological*. The two are not the same. The child may well be abnormal in the statistical sense, but otherwise quite healthy. It will be up to the pediatrician to determine if there is anything else in the history or physical exam that would suggest pathology.

The situation is even worse when the parent does not even know the range of normal, but only the mean weight, or age at which a child first sits up. She may think her child is clinically abnormal sitting up at 7 months rather than the mean of 6, even though the child may be quite healthy.

As another example, the normal range of intraocular pressure is about 10–20 mmHg. Above that number, there is an increasing possibility that the patient may develop glaucoma, a disease in which high pressure in the eye causes blindness. What if the patient has a pressure of 26? That is clearly abnormal in the statistical sense. Should the doctor immediately start the patient on glaucoma drops for *the rest of the patient's life*? The wise physician knows that the abnormal pressure may be abnormal only in the statistical sense; there are patients who have pressures in the 30s yet never run into trouble (just are there are patients with pressures in the teens who may develop glaucoma). People with high intraocular pressures are abnormal statistically but may be normal clinically. Rather than put this "abnormal" patient immediately on lifetime eye drops, the correct approach is to follow the patient every 6 months or so to see if there are any beginning signs of glaucoma; if there are, then start the patient on medication.

The confusion between statistical and clinical abnormality came to public focus with the Kinsey report on teens and premarital sex. When Dr. Kinsey indicated that certain practices were "normal," some people thought he meant that these practices were OK to do, and attacked him on moral grounds. However, the "normal" he mentioned was statistical, which offers no opinion as to right or wrong.

CHAPTER 2. MEAN, MEDIAN, AND MODE

The word "average" has different meanings. It can refer to *mean*, *median*, or *mode*.

Mean

Consider the series of 8 numbers:

1, 10, 20, 30, 40, 47, 47, 50

The (arithmetic) **mean** is obtained by adding up the numbers and dividing by the total number (N) of numbers:

$$\frac{(1 + 10 + 20 + 30 + 40 + 47 + 47 + 50)}{8} = 30.63$$

Median

The **median** (like the "median" in a highway) is simply the center number in the ordered sequence of data points. If there is an odd number of digits, the median is the center number. If there is an even number of digits, the median is halfway between the two central numbers (35 in this case).

Mode

The **mode** (sounds like "most") is the number that appears most often in the sequence (47 here). If there is no mode, the data is **amodal**. Sometimes there may be two or more modes, in which case the data is **bimodal**, **trimodal**, etc. (**Fig. 2–1**).

The (arithmetic) mean is the most common way to describe an "average." It takes every number into account. However, it has its drawbacks. Sometimes the data is very skewed, because there is one or a few values, termed **outliers**, that are very far off the chart. Averaging them in, using a mean, can be very deceptive. For instance consider the same number sequence as above, but with 500 at the end instead of 50:

1 10 20 30 40 47 47 500

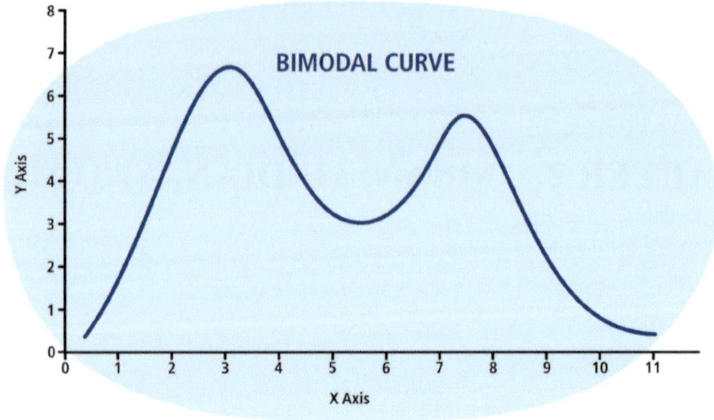

Figure 2–1. Bimodal curve.

Then, the mean jumps up to 86.88, while the median and mode remain unchanged and are more useful descriptions of the average when the curve is non-normal. The mean moves in the direction of outliers.

A **trimmed mean** is one in which the highest and lowest values are omitted, thus reducing the distorting effect of outliers. A *5% trimmed mean* is one in which the top 5% and lowest 5% of data are removed.

A **weighted mean (overall mean)** is a mean combined from several samples of different sizes. Larger samples are given more weight than smaller samples. Thus, each mean is multiplied by its **n** (total number in the sample), all the products are summed, and then divided by the total **N** (number of data points in the entire dataset).

An **approximate mean** resembles the weighted mean, but is used where data points are in intervals (such as 1–10, 11–20, etc.). The midpoint of each interval is multiplied by the interval's **n** (number of data points in the interval), all these are summed, and then divided by **N** (total number of data points in the study).

A **geometric mean (GM)** summarizes change over time as the average ratio or rate of change, for example in tracking how fast a medical practice grew. Say the practice served 1000, 3000, and 7000 patients over 3 years. Patient load tripled from year 1 to year 2 (3000/1000 = 3) and increased 2.33 from year 2 to year 3 (7000/3000 = 2.33). Here, calculate the geometric mean (GM) by multiplying the rates of change together and taking the root of the product. In this example, we multiply 3 × 2.33 = 7. Since we multiplied two numbers, we'll take the square root of seven, which equals 2.65. GM = 2.65. The practice load increased by an average factor of 2.65 each year. The root (square root, cube root, etc.) depends on how many data points are being averaged (n). Use the nth root. When n = 2, use the square root of the product of the multiplications. When n = 3, use the cube root of the product; if n = 4, use the 4th root, etc.

A geometric mean is commonly used when the study involves exponential growth (e.g. bacterial colonies, radioactive decay, drug half-life), or when the data for gains and losses is presented as a percentage.

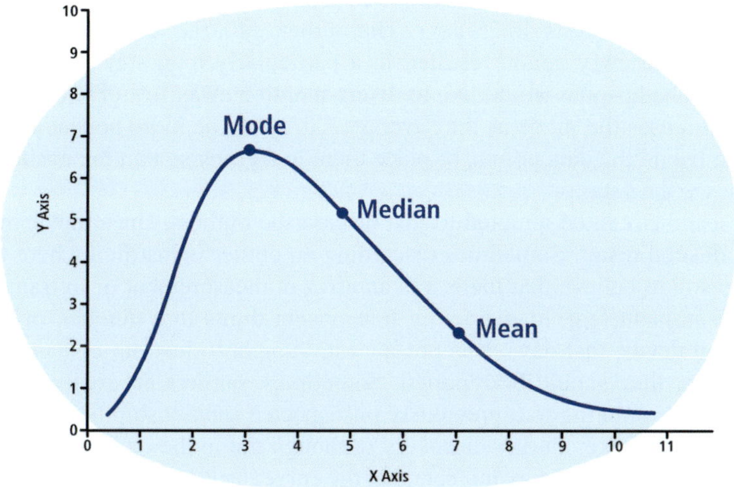

Figure 2–2. Positioning of mean, median, and mode on data with positive skew. The positions of the mode and mean are switched on data with negative skew.

In describing an "average," the median is often a better choice than the mode, since there may not even be a mode if all the data points are different, or there may be two or more modes. Sometimes a mode, though, may provide useful information. For instance, a bimodal curve may appear when combining the information from two different groups, such as the heights of women and men of a certain age, all combined. The curve would be bimodal, showing two peaks, one reflecting the heights of women and the other of men. Just reporting the mean or median would miss this. Sometimes the appearance of a bimodal or trimodal curve is unexpected and provides new information.

Whenever a report mentions an average, it is important to be clear whether this is the mean, median, mode, or another kind of average.

In a symmetrical curve, the mean, median, and mode are the same. If there is skew, the mode, of course, will still be the highest point on the curve, but the mean and median will be shifted so that the median is in the "middle" between the mode and mean. The mean will lie on the outermost portion of the curve (**Fig. 2–2**). One way to tell if a curve is reasonably normal is to see if the mean and median are reasonably close. A more precise way is to see if the skew is 2.0 or less. (The math for determining this is beyond the scope of this book. Leave that to the biostatisticians and computer software.)

What's Wrong Here? *#!!

A hospital reports that its "average hospital stay is 3 days." *What's wrong?*: An unqualified "average" is almost pointless. Consider the following times in days of patient stays:

1 3 3 3 5 6 9 340

The hospital has reported the mode (3 days). If the "average" refers to the mean, then the average stay is 46.25 days. The outlier, 340, the result of Dr. Nerdly's operation gone awry again, resulted in a particularly long stay and throws off the mean. The hospital would like to divert attention away from Dr. Nerdly's bad results, and uses the mode as the "average." It would be more honest and meaningful to list all the data points, or place them in a graph so that the evaluator can directly see the data.

A researcher can be tempted to just discard the outliers, since they can throw off the desired result. Sometimes discarding an outlier is justified where there is good reason to believe that there was an error in measurement or in transcribing the measurement (e.g. inadvertently transposing digits in a number, or a faulty measuring device that day). It is not honest, though, to just out-of-hand dismiss the outliers; they should be reported. Sometimes, outliers are really significant new findings, pointing to a previously unsuspected relationship; one could get a Nobel Prize for a key outlier discovery (although not in the case of Dr. Nerdly!). At other times, outliers may indicate that the curve itself is not Gaussian. The data in the curve may, for instance, be distributed in a *lognormal* distribution, namely one in which the data can be transformed to a Gaussian distribution by taking the logarithm (**Fig. 2–3**). If the curves can't be converted, a nonparametric statistical method may need to be used (**Chapter 17**).

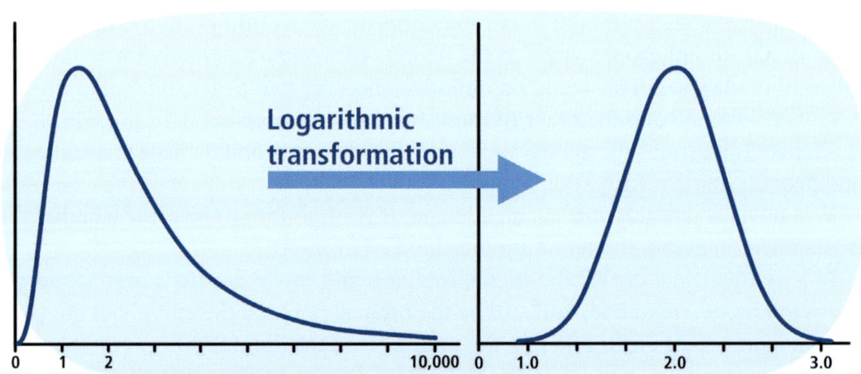

Figure 2–3. Logarithmic transformation to a Gaussian curve.

CHAPTER 3. RANGE, VARIANCE, AND STANDARD DEVIATION

A bell-shaped curve is defined not only by its mean, median, and mode, but also by the degree of dispersion of its data. The curves in **Fig. 3–1**, for instance, have the same mean, median, and mode. However, the dispersion of points (scatter) in curve B is wider than in curve A.

Range

A simple way to describe this spread is the **range**, namely the difference between the highest and lowest values. Range, though, has limitations. Examples:

1. Family practitioners may see a range of 8 patients per day (min = 52, max = 60), and plastic surgeons may also see a range of 8 patients per day (min = 1, max = 9). This shows that similar ranges may correspond to very different workloads, a point missed on simply stating the range.
2. Three students whose test scores are shown below all have a range of 49 points, but the distribution of the data reveals dramatic differences in how they have performed:

Lin: 1, 2, 4, 6, 8, 10, 12, 50
Lindsay: 1, 10, 20, 30, 40, 47, 50, 50
Laurie: 1, 43, 43, 44, 45, 46, 47, 50

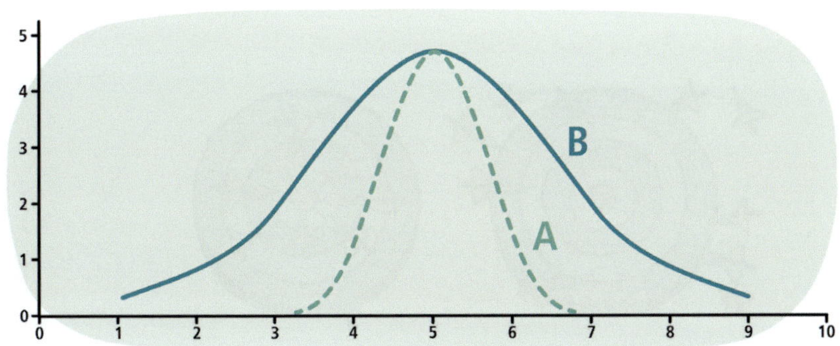

Figure 3–1. Curves A and B have the same mean, median, and mode, but curve A has less scatter (dispersion) than curve B.

Variance

A more detailed way of describing the spread is **variance** (think of it as "variability among the data points"). The formula for variance is:

$$\text{Variance} = \frac{\sum(X-\underline{M})2}{n-1}$$

where
$\sum$ = the sum of
X = the data point (element)
$\underline{M}$ = the group's mean
n = the number of data points (elements) in the group. (Sometimes N, rather than n, is used, particularly when N refers to the number in the population.)

Standard Deviation

The **standard deviation (SD)**, which is a more intuitive concept than the variance, is the square root of variance. **Fig. 3–2** shows a useful metaphor for standard deviation. If the bull's-eye is the mean and the darts are individual data points, standard deviation is the average distance between the data points and the mean. There is greater variability in the "data" on the dartboard on the left, illustrated by the greater scatter of the "darts" around the bull's-eye, in contrast with the dartboard on the right.

Don't panic over the math. We won't go into the derivation of the formulae for variance and standard deviation. Just note here that the numerator involves the differences between the elements of the curve and the curve's mean. The greater those differences, the greater the spread of data in the standard deviation.

Sometimes researchers report what the variance is rather than the standard deviation, and variance plays a role in the calculations of a number of equations in biostatistics. It is easier, though, to picture what a standard deviation of 10 mmHg means than to picture what a variance of $(10\ \text{mmHg})^2$ means.

In a normal (Gaussian) curve, about 68% of the data points of the curve lie within what is called one **standard deviation** on either side of the mean (**Fig. 3–3**). About 95% of data points lie within 2 (actually 1.96) standard deviations from the mean and

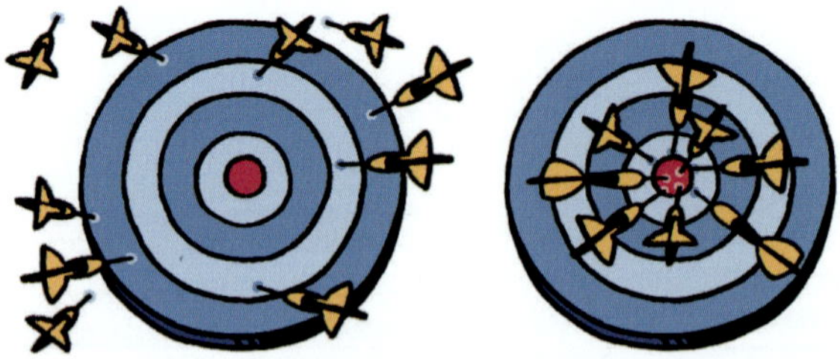

Figure 3–2. Dartboard analogy for Standard Deviation. From Weaver, A., 2005.

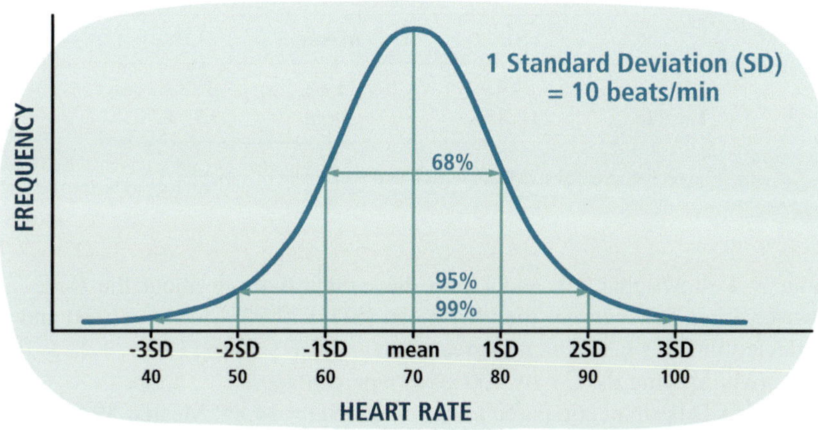

Figure 3–3. The 68-95-99 rule for a Gaussian curve: 68% of the area of the curve lies within 1 standard deviation from the mean; 95% lies within 2 standard deviations; 99% lies within 3 standard deviations.

about 99% (actually 99.7%) lie within 3 standard deviations (the "68-95-99 rule") (**Fig. 3–3**). Standard deviation is a measure of the spread of the data. Thin curves, which have less variability in the data, have smaller standard deviations; wider curves have larger SDs. A **z-score** is the number of standard deviations a data point (element) lies away from the mean.

For instance, **Fig. 3–3** plots heart rate in beats per minute. This population has a mean of 70 beats/min and a standard deviation of 10 beats/min. 90 beats per minute is a data point that lies 2 standard deviations from the mean according to the simple formula:

$$z = \frac{\text{(the data point} - \text{population mean)}}{\text{population standard deviation}}$$

$$2 = (90 - 70)/10$$

Mean and standard deviation can be determined from data that don't fall in a Gaussian distribution, but if the curve isn't normal (Gaussian), you can't use z-scores or the 68-95-99 rule.

If you know the mean and standard deviation, you know essentially all the points in a normal (Gaussian) curve.

Coefficient of Variation

Coefficient of Variation (CV) = SD/Mean

CV is another way of looking at the scatter of data points around the mean. For example, recall the grade scores for Lin and Laurie:

Lin: 1, 2, 4, 6, 8, 10, 12, 50

Laurie: 1, 43, 43, 44, 45, 46, 47, 50

	SD	Mean	CV
Lin	14.93	11.63	128%
Laurie	14.85	39.88	37%

Figure 3–4. Standard deviation (SD) and coefficient of variation (CV).

Fig. 3–4 shows that Lin and Laurie have SDs that are about the same size. However, Lin's SD is *larger* than her mean (SD = 14.93; Mean = 11.63) and this is reflected in Lin's CV, which is greater than 100% (14.93/11.63 = 1.28 × 100 = 128%). (Multiplying the CV by 100 gives a percentage.)

Laurie's CD is small compared to her mean (SD = 14.85; Mean = 39.88); this is reflected in Laurie's small CV of 37%. This is because the variability of Laurie's data relative to the mean is less than that of Lin, even though their SDs are close. Lin's scatter is greater than that of Laurie. So CV is a valuable way of describing scatter.

Another value to the coefficient of variation: When SD is divided by the mean, the units (e.g. weight, height, age, lab value, etc.) cancel out, and the result is a pure number. This can make it easier to compare variations in two studies, each of which may have the same results, but use different units of measure. Similarly, while SD is described in units, a z-score is described in number of standard deviations, and can be used to compare two studies that use different units of measure.

CHAPTER 4. KINDS OF DATA

Nominal Data

Nominal data are categories in *name* only, with no particular order, e.g. blood types A, B, AB, and O are nominal data. It makes no difference how you order them, whether (A, B, AB, O) or (B, A, O, AB). If there were 10 people with blood type A, 7 with B, 4 with AB, and 8 with O, for instance, there can be a *mode* (the 10 A's being most common) but no mean (what would be the average between an A and a B?), and no median, since the data are not in any particular order.

Ordinal Data

Ordinal data are like nominal data but follow a particular *order* (e.g. pain on a scale of 1 to 5). Since ordinal data are ordered, both *median* and *mode* can be used to describe ordinal data. Often the mean is not appropriate for describing this data, since it is not clear that the difference between a 1 and a 2 on a pain scale is the same quantitative difference as the difference between a 2 and a 3, for instance, so what would a mean of 2.3 really mean? However, if the differences between categories are considered to be equal, you can use a *mean* for ordinal data.

Interval Data

Interval data are like ordinal data in that they can be placed in a clear order, but also have clear set quantitative differences between the numbers. For instance, temperatures, whether in Fahrenheit or Centigrade, are interval data; the difference between 5 °F and 4 °F is the same difference as between 60 °F and 59 °F. Interval data, however, do not have a meaningful zero; zero degrees F does not mean "no temperature." 100 °F is not twice as hot as 50 °F (consider the temperature of boiling water and ice, which are respectively 212 °F and 32 °F, versus 100 °C and 0 °C); the boiling/freezing ratio in °F is not comparable to that in °C. It is meaningful to describe *intervals* of interval data (e.g. 100°F minus 50°F = 50 °F), as well as means involving the data (e.g. "average temperature was (100 °F plus 50 °F)/2 = 75 °F") but not *ratios* between the data (e.g.100°F/50°F). You can describe interval data with either a *mean*, *median* or *mode*.

Ratio Data

Ratio data are like interval data, but *can* be reported as ratios, since ratio data have a meaningful zero. For instance, the range of scores on an exam (e.g. 40, 60, 75, 80, 90, 95) can be described not only as intervals (90 is 5 points higher than 85), but also as ratios (someone with an 80 did twice as well as someone with 40), since there can be a meaningful "0"(!). Like interval data, ratio data can be described with a *mean*, *median*, or *mode*.

Nominal and ordinal data are termed **categorical** (or **nonmetric**) **data**. They are categories (**Fig. 4–1**).

Interval and ratio data are termed **numeric** (or **metric**) **data** and can be either **discrete** or **continuous data**. **Discrete data** are whole numbers, without intermediary values, e.g. the number of people or observations (there cannot be 5.2 observations). **Continuous data** can have intermediary values, such as temperature (for instance 99.6 °F).

Interval and ratio data (and sometimes ordinal data) have a *mean*, *median*, *mode*, and *standard deviation*, and commonly follow a *Gaussian distribution*. When all these are the case, **parametric statistics** can be used to evaluate such data.

Nominal data can have a mode, but no median, mean or standard deviation. Such data do not fit a Gaussian distribution.

Ordinal data can have a median and a mode (but generally not a mean or standard deviation) (**Fig. 4–1**). Thus, **nonparametric statistics** are used to deal with nominal and ordinal data (**Chapter 17**). Note, however, that an increasing number of biostatisticians grant the use of parametric statistics on ordinal data when those data are Gaussian.

Measurement Scales of Data	
CATEGORICAL (Nonmetric)	**NUMERIC (Metric)**
Unordered (Nominal) Data: • e.g. ABO blood grouping • Use the mode for analysis	**Interval Data:** • Has no meaningful absolute zero, e.g. Fahrenheit or Celcius temperature • Use the mean, median, or mode for analysis
Ordered (Ordinal) Data: • e.g. Rating pain from 1 to 5 • Use the mode, median, and sometimes the mean for analysis	**Ratio Data:** • Has a meaningful absolute zero, e.g. exam grades • Use the mean, median, or mode for analysis

Figure 4–1. Measurement scales of data.

PART II
RESEARCH DESIGN

CHAPTER 5. KINDS OF STUDIES

Randomized Control Studies

Rather than just testing a potentially useful analgesic and recording the percentage of people who report a lessening of pain, it is important to have **controls**, patients who receive a placebo rather than the drug. Patients often report improvement with placebos, so adding the placebo control tells the researcher whether the drug effect is better than that of the placebo, and by how much. It is important in controlled studies to *match* the drug and control groups for age, sex, disease severity, occupation, and other factors. Otherwise, an improvement might be due to factors other than the treatment itself. Randomization of subjects is not an issue when the controls are the same people: comparing the patient before and after the treatment, or using the right and left sides of the patient's body, one side for the treatment and the other side without.

It is important to understand that there are two kinds of randomization processes:

1. Randomly selecting people from the population. The sample of people in the study should be *representative of the population* and not biased.
2. Once the people have been randomly selected, they must *be randomly assigned to groups*, either treatment(s) or control. It is easier to do the latter than to randomly select from the population without bias, but it can be problematic if the researcher puts people more likely to improve, or in worse shape, into the treatment group. So when the researcher states that the participants were "randomly selected," what does this mean? Randomly selected from the population, or randomly divided into two groups? This has to be made clear.

Matching Studies

Rather than simply selecting people randomly for an experimental and control group, selection can be done by purposefully **matching** people for such variables as age, sex, severity of disease, or race.

Stratified Randomization Studies

Stratified randomization is a mixture of matching and simple randomization. For instance, if you were testing the effect of a new drug on urinary frequency in men ages 66–75 versus those ages 76–85, first **stratify** the population into two groups, 66–75 and 76–85 year-old men. Then **randomly** select people from the stratified groups to include in either the treatment or control groups.

Blind Studies

Ideally, comparing a treatment with a placebo or with an alternative treatment should be done in the blind. In the **double-blind** method, neither the physician nor patient knows which treatment the patient is getting until the results are in. This prevents bias on the part of the patient and physician in evaluating the treatment's effect. It is not always possible to hide from the patient or physician whether it is treatment or control, which may be the case when the treatment is surgery, or the drug has very noticeable systemic effects.

Prospective (Cohort; Longitudinal) Studies

In **prospective** (**cohort**) studies, the results of the treatment or other intervention are not known until some time after the intervention. Prospective studies can be used to follow what happens to patients who have received a particular treatment or who have been exposed to a risk factor, such as radiation.

For instance, in evaluating whether an antiarrhythmic drug decreases sudden cardiac deaths, patients are given either the drug or control, and are then followed over a number of years to determine which group has the greatest incidence of death. Such studies can be long and expensive, however, particularly if the disease rarely appears, in which case large numbers of people may be necessary for the study. The researcher may opt to instead use a **surrogate (proxy)** end point, such as whether the drug reduces arrhythmias. Since arrhythmias are correlated with sudden death, presumably a reduction of arrhythmias will also decrease the number of sudden deaths. This approach is risky, because it may not be known if the drug has side effects that over months or years may in fact *increase* the risk of death. It also presumes that the arrhythmias cause the sudden death. That may not be the case. Instead, the correlation between arrhythmias and sudden death may be the opposite: that a damaged heart causes the arrhythmias, rather than the arrhythmias causing the deaths. Treating the arrhythmia may then do no good, but leave the subject susceptible to side effects of the treatment. This problem, in fact, did occur in the 1980's (Moore, '95), when antiarrhythmics were widely prescribed, even for non-life threatening arrhythmias, leading to many unnecessary deaths (which initially were felt to be due to the heart disease, rather than the drugs), until studies were properly done to assess whether the drugs actually saved lives. They didn't; they killed thousands of people. Thus, it is important in doing a prospective study to note whether the study is trying to evaluate the main question ("Does the treatment prevent death?"), or does the study use a surrogate (proxy) question ("Does the treatment reduce arrhythmias?").

Laboratory tests are commonly used as surrogates. Trying to treat an illness by improving the value of a laboratory test may not necessarily improve health. Sometimes, it works, though, e.g. trying to increase CD4+ counts in HIV. Other times, surrogates don't work. For example, serum homocysteine is correlated with cardiovascular disease, but reducing homocysteine doesn't help. Perhaps homocysteine is just a marker of cardiovascular disease, not a cause. Perhaps cardiovascular disease causes a rise in homocysteine, not the opposite; or perhaps a third factor causes both a rise in homocysteine and cardiovascular disease. Correlation does not prove causation.

PROS of prospective studies:

- They can use random sampling.
- They can provide good information about risk.

CONS of prospective studies:

- They can take a long time.
- They can be expensive.
- Patients may be lost to follow-up by the researcher.

Examples of questions amenable to prospective studies:

- Do cardiac stents save lives?
- Does prayer contribute to recovery?
- Does treatment of hypertension or elevated cholesterol reduce the incidence of cardiovascular disease?
- Do silicon breast implants cause immune diseases?
- Does estrogen supplementation cause breast cancer?
- Are specific vitamins or diets helpful for specific conditions?
- Does decreasing serum homocysteine save lives?
- Do Class I antiarrhythmics save lives?
- Do drugs for Alzheimer's disease, including those to reduce cerebral plaques, improve mental functioning? (Do cerebral plaques cause Alzheimer's disease, or does Alzheimer's disease cause plaques?)
- Does estrogen administration reduce cardiovascular disease?
- Does blood sugar stabilization lessen the likelihood of cardiovascular disease in diabetics?
- How effective is screening for breast cancer, lung cancer, colon cancer, or prostate cancer?

Retrospective (Case-Control) Studies

When the condition of interest is rare, it can be very difficult to perform a prospective study. A **retrospective study** collects patients who have the condition and looks for potential risk factors in their past. For instance, *phocomelia* (infants born with limbs that look like flippers) is rare. A retrospective study discovered that a high percentage of mothers of these children had taken the drug *thalidomide* during pregnancy. This led to the discontinuation of the drug.

Retrospective studies may rely on patient recall, medical records, or autopsy.

PROS of retrospective studies:

- This research method is more ethical, not purposefully exposing a patient to a potential risk factor.
- It is less expensive and less time-consuming than prospective studies.
- The researcher can consult past records and study multiple potential causes of the disease.
- Retrospective studies are better than prospective studies in studying rare diseases.

CONS of retrospective studies:

- Bias. They are not double blind, and they may rely on patient recall, which often is faulty. Patients with the disease are more likely to think about what may have caused the disease than controls. One retrospective study suggested that women who had abortions were more likely to get breast cancer. The study presumes that both the study and control group answered the survey with the same degree of honesty, which is not necessarily so. Healthy people may be less likely to admit to an abortion than sick people, who may be more likely to be forthright about their past medical history.
- It may be hard to select a matching control group. (In the case of phocomelia, though, the findings were so obvious that a control group was unnecessary.)

Examples of questions amenable to retrospective studies:

- Does estrogen supplementation increase the incidence of breast cancer?
- Does smoking cause lung cancer?
- Does asbestos cause mesothelioma?
- Are high tension wires, cell phones, or microwave ovens associated with an increased incidence of leukemia or brain cancer?
- Do vaccines cause autism?
- Do sunlight and tanning salons contribute to skin cancer?

Cross-Sectional (Prevalence) Studies

As opposed to prospective and retrospective studies, which look at individuals over a period of time, **cross-sectional studies** look at a group of people at a given slice of time. For instance, the study may issue a questionnaire to determine what fraction of a population at a given time wears a hearing aid or has a particular opinion about abortion.

Questions not infrequently arise as to the origin of cancer clusters in a particular small town (e.g. 10 children in the town developed a rare brain cancer within a short time). Here, we not only have to compare the prevalence of the cancer in the affected town with the prevalence in other towns, but consider the question of whether the prevalence in the affected town is coincidental. Of thousands of kinds of uncommon diseases, the chances are reasonably high that one of them will by chance arise in a particular town. Also, of thousands of towns, there is a likelihood that one of them by chance will have a particular rare disease cluster. It may be necessary to follow up and determine whether the incidence continues to be high, in addition to searching for a toxic influence.

PROS of cross-sectional studies:

- They are cheaper and easier to perform than longitudinal studies.
- Follow-up is commonly unnecessary.

CONS of cross-sectional studies:

- They can tell us about prevalence of a condition (i.e. the number of people who have the condition at a particular time), but not the incidence (what percentage of people will acquire the condition within a year).
- Surveys can be very susceptible to bias. Not everyone chooses to answer a survey. Moreover, the questions themselves may be biased. For instance, consider the likely difference in responses to the following alternative survey questions:

a. How do you feel about killing unborn babies?
b. How do you feel about forced continuation of pregnancy?

You have to ask, "Is the survey designed to *discover* public opinion or to *shape* public opinion?"

Experimental vs. Observational Studies

In an **experimental study**, the investigator randomly divides a sample of people into two groups, one of which receives the treatment or risk factor, while the other receives an alternative treatment (or a placebo), and compares the results. For instance, to assess the effect of smoking on lung vital capacity, one group would be assigned cigarettes to smoke heavily for 10 years, and a matched group would not. The vital capacity of each group would then be determined (followed by the lawsuits against the researchers).

PROS of experimental studies:

- They can be used to evaluate a new treatment, for which there is no data as yet.
- They can verify a previous finding, or evaluate the new treatment on a different group of patients (e.g. different gender, age, or ethnicity).

CONS of experimental studies:

- It can be unethical to expose patients to a risk factor.
- They can be time-consuming and expensive.

In an **observational study**, the investigator observes the patients, collecting data about them without assigning any treatment or risk factor to them. The investigator finds a group of patients who have smoked for 10 years and compares their vital capacity to a matched group of nonsmokers. Observational studies can be prospective or retrospective.

PROS of observational studies:

- There is no ethical problem, since the researcher does not purposely introduce the risk factor.

CONS of observational studies:

- The investigator has no control over how the treatment or risk factor is delivered. This lack of control can introduce variability that may mask the true effect of the risk factor.

Case Series and Case Reports

Both the case series and case report can provide information about rare occurrences.

A **case series** describes a number of patients with an unusual disease presentation, sometimes involving patients a physician has encountered over years in practice, or collected from the literature. A **case report** is the description of a *single* patient.

Meta-Analysis

Sometimes a single research study does not provide enough information. In a **meta-analysis** the researcher searches the literature and combines the information from a number of studies.

PROS of meta-analysis:

- By combining studies, meta-analysis can produce an adequate sample size to study.
- Meta-analysis also can point to the variability of the effect of the independent variable (e.g. the treatment) in the different studies.

CONS of meta-analysis:

- Meta-analysis relies on published studies and cannot control for poor studies, bias, and design differences among the combined studies.

Crossover, Between-Subjects, and Within-Subjects Studies

Between-subjects studies compare one group of patients with another.

Within-subjects studies compare one group of patients with itself, e.g. a before-and-after picture. Within-subjects studies have the advantage of automatically eliminating confounding group differences that might be present when the groups differ.

Cross-over studies combine the between-subject and within-subject formats. One group receives the treatment followed (after a "washout" period to rule out a persisting drug effect) by a placebo (within-subjects). A comparable group does the same thing, but in reverse, receiving the placebo first and then the treatment (within-subjects). Then the two group results are compared (between-subjects). This counterbalancing of the sequence of presentation of treatment and placebo helps to confirm whether or not having the placebo before or after alters the result.

Therapeutic Trials

In order to save time and expense, and guard against the potential for adverse effects, therapeutic trials are commonly divided into 4 phases:

Phase I: The treatment is given to a small number of people (commonly 20–50), often healthy volunteers, but sometimes patients, to look at the safety of the drug and its pharmacokinetics.

Phase II: The treatment is given to a larger group of patients (often 50–300), noting treatment effectiveness and adverse effects, and fine-tuning the dosage.

Phase III: A larger study is used (300–3,000 or more), comparing patients with controls who take a placebo or a competing treatment.

Phase IV: After the drug has been approved and gone to market, phase IV follows up to see if there are any rare or long-term adverse effects or interactions with other drugs.

CHAPTER 6. KINDS OF GRAPHS

Bar Graphs (Bar Charts)

If the data are nominal or ordinal, they can be shown as bar graphs (bar charts), in which the bars do not have touching sides (**Fig. 6–1A**). The sides are separated (like stools in a *bar*), so that the viewer does not mistakenly think they are a continuous sequence; they are separate categories.

It can be deceiving if bar charts or other graphs do not start their y axis at 0, as is correctly done in **Fig. 6–1A**. In **Fig. 6–1B**, hospital administrator Bob Gnarley, in a ploy to try to convince the Board to hire more oncologists and cardiologists, redid the graph so that the y axis didn't start at 0 physicians. Instead, it started at 20. This made it visually appear as if the hospital was short of oncologists and cardiologists. This is a common error. It can be checked through the **Graph Discrepancy Index (GDI)**, which detects faulty axis distortions:

$$\textbf{GDI} = \frac{\text{Percentage rise in the graph height}}{\text{Percentage rise in the data}} - 1$$

For perfect proportional graphics, the GDI should equal 0, although a GDI no higher than 0.5 is considered acceptable. In **Fig. 6–1A**, the percentage difference in the height of the cardiologist bar as compared with the general practitioner bar is about 175% (from 20 to 35 physicians, the same as the data (20 × 1.75 = 35). So the GDI is (1.75/1.75) – 1 = 0. However in **Fig. 6–1B**, the general practitioner

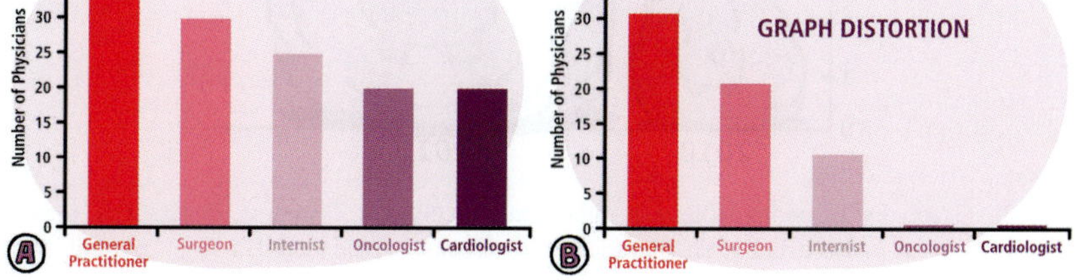

Figure 6–1. Graph distortion, by failing to set the baseline at 0.

bar is about 30 times higher than the cardiologist bar, so the DGI is 30/1.75 = 17.4. For shame!

Hospital administrator Gnarly also visually exaggerated his hospital's profits through a 3 dimensional graph (**Fig. 6–2**). The profits doubled (correctly), as indicated by the heights of the money bags. However, the width of the bags also doubled, looking like a quadruple change in profits. It is best to avoid 3D graphs.

Tables

You can show data in different ways. One way is to just list all the numbers in a **table**. If there are too many numbers to list in a table, you can list the data as ranges of numbers, called **intervals** (**Fig. 6–3**). It is often most helpful, though, to show the data in a graph (**Fig. 6–4**).

Histograms

A **histogram** is used for interval or ratio data. The data are commonly presented as bars reflecting a series of intervals (**Fig. 6–4**). The sequence of intervals is plotted on the graph as rectangles, whose sides touch one another, since this is continuous data. (There may, however, be a gap between certain bars where a given interval of data points is missing.) The researcher has to decide how wide

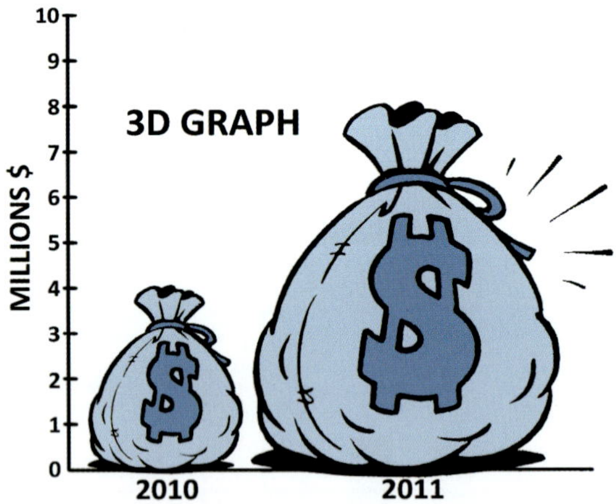

Figure 6–2. Graph distortion, by using 3D, rather than 2D, figures. The money in 2011 is supposed to be twice as much as in 2010, but looks like four times as much, since the 2011 bag is not only twice as high, but twice as wide as the bag in 2010.

Hypothetical Data on Serum Uric Acid Levels			
Uric Acid Levels (mg/dl)	**Number of Donors**	**Cumulative Frequencies**	**Cumulative Percents**
3.0–3.9	40	40	31%
4.0–4.9	30	70	54%
5.0–5.9	25	95	73%
6.0–6.9	20	115	88%
7.0–7.9	10	125	96%
8.0–8.9	5	130	100%
	N = 130		

Figure 6–3.

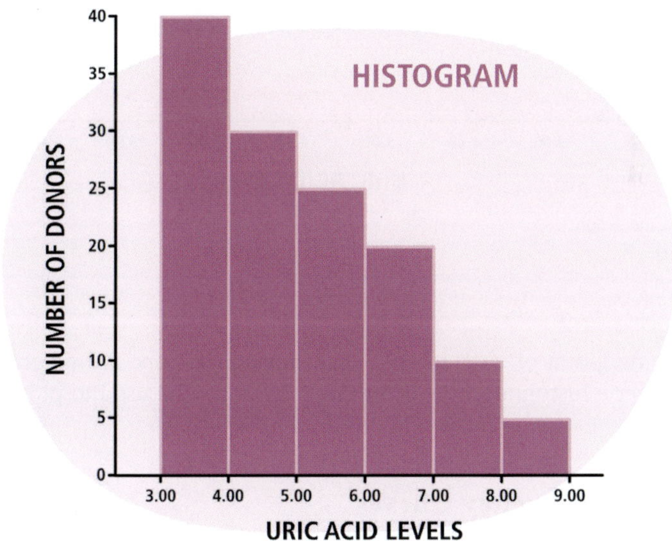

Figure 6–4. Histogram.

the intervals should be (e.g. "1–10, 11–20" vs. "1–5, 6–10, 11–15, 16–20," etc.). The data can be difficult to read when there are too many bars. With too few bars, information is lost.

Line Graphs

For interval or ratio data, you can use a **line graph**, in which each bar's midpoint is connected to the next by a straight line (**Fig. 6–5**). Since histograms represent continuous data, they can be converted into line graphs by "connecting the

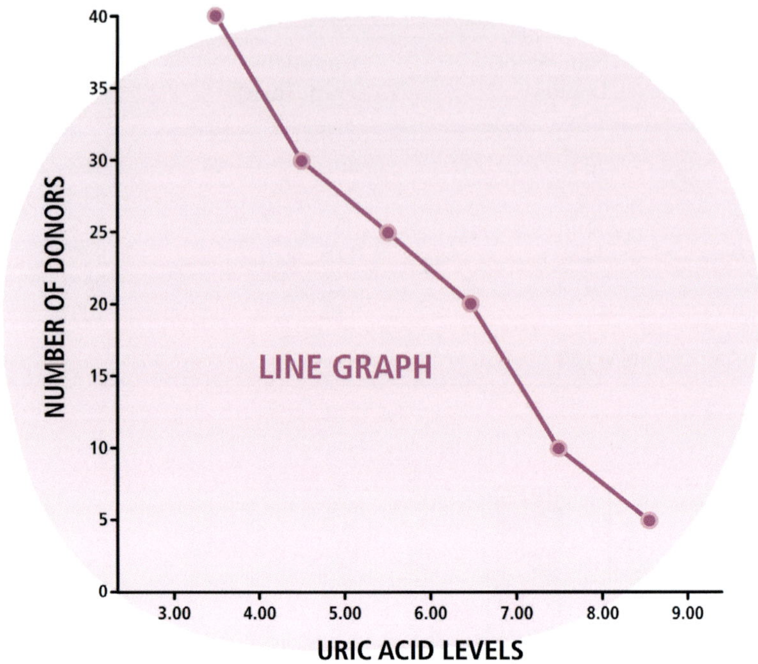

Figure 6–5. Line graph.

dots" at the midpoint of each interval and erasing the bars. A line graph has an advantage over a histogram in that the same chart can be used to plot more than one group.

Cumulative Frequency Curves

In a **cumulative frequency curve**, the frequency of each data point is successively added to the previous frequency, proceeding from left to right. The ordinate (y axis) of such a graph thus plots the data from 0 to 100%. For instance, compare **Fig. 6–3** with **Fig. 6–6**. They both have the same information. The frequencies of all the data points always add up to 100%. Frequency distributions can be graphed as a line or histogram, or presented as a table.

The line graph symbolizing a cumulative frequency or percent distribution is called an **ogive** ("g" pronounced like "j")(**Fig. 6–6**). An ogive has an S-shape when the data is Gaussian (**Fig. 6–7**) and can be useful, for instance, in quickly determining what data point lies at the 90th percentile, or what percentile corresponds to a given data value.

Question: For diseases on the rise, like AIDS, would a histogram or an ogive be a better way to represent rate of increase over time?

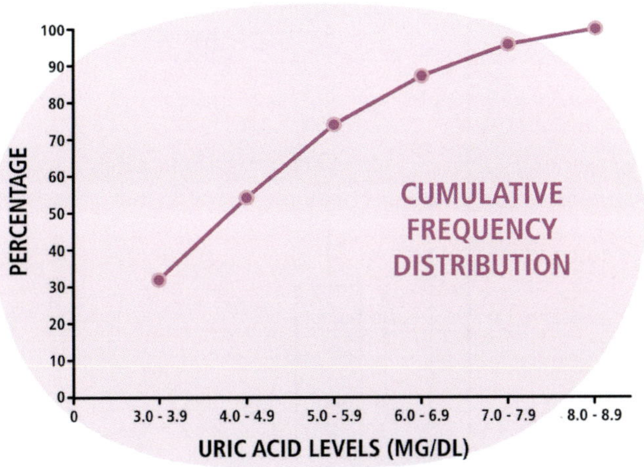

Figure 6–6. Cumulative frequency distribution graph of uric acid levels.

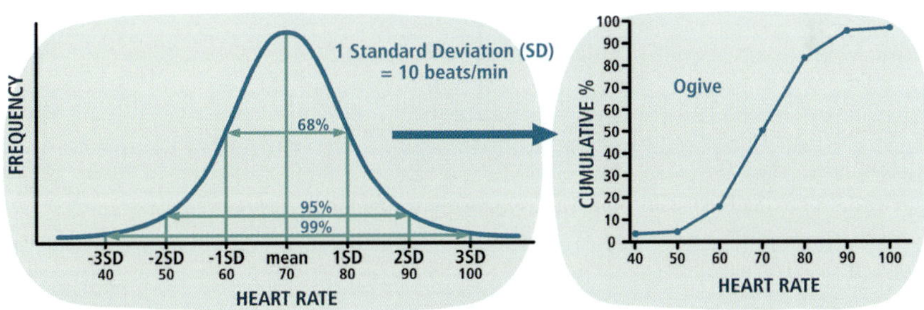

Figure 6–7. Conversion of a Gaussian curve to an ogive.

Answer: Ogive. This kind of graph is designed to show *rates of change* over time, revealed by how steeply the line on the graph rises across units of time, and if/how/when it begins to level out. In the AIDS example, the y axis would be labeled from 0 to 100% and the x axis labeled "Year" in an ogive. In contrast, the y axis would be labeled "Number of Cases" and the x axis labeled "Year" in the histogram, which would not show the rate of increase.

Box-and-Whiskers Plots

A **box-and-whiskers plot**, as shown in **Fig. 6–8**, can present a lot of information at a glance. The rectangular area (**interquartile range**) represents where the middle 50% of the data can be found, stretching from the 25th to the

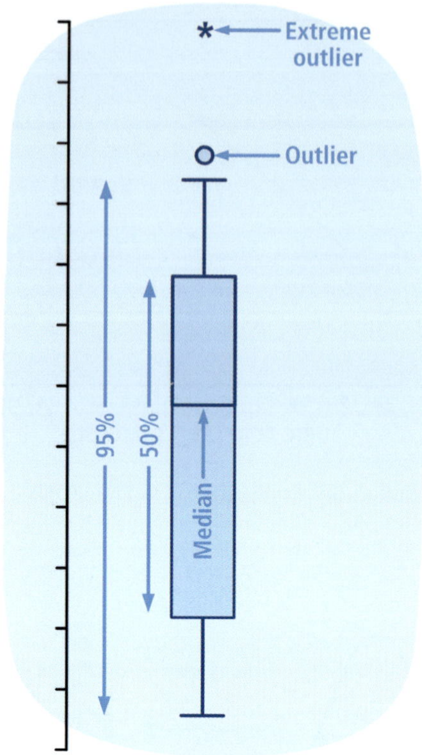

Figure 6–8. A box-and-whiskers plot. The asymmetric median indicates skewed data.

75th percentile. The whiskers that protrude from either side commonly span the 95% range of the data, but they can be drawn to span the entire range of data. The line inside the rectangle shows the median of the data. An asymmetric median indicates skew. Outliers are indicated by points outside the whiskers, a circle commonly used to indicate a relatively close outlier (commonly 1.5–3 times the length of the box), and an asterisk for an extreme outlier (commonly more than 3 times the length of the box).

Stem-and-Leaf Plots

A **stem-and-leaf plot** shows the maximum information, by showing each data point. The leftmost column (in bold in **Fig. 6–9**) is the stem, which lists the "tens" digits vertically. The "leaves" are the "ones" digits, in the rows to the right of the "tens" numbers. If you turn a stem-and-leaf plot sideways, it forms a histogram. **Fig. 6–9** then resembles **Fig. 6–4**, except that **Fig. 6–9** contains more information.

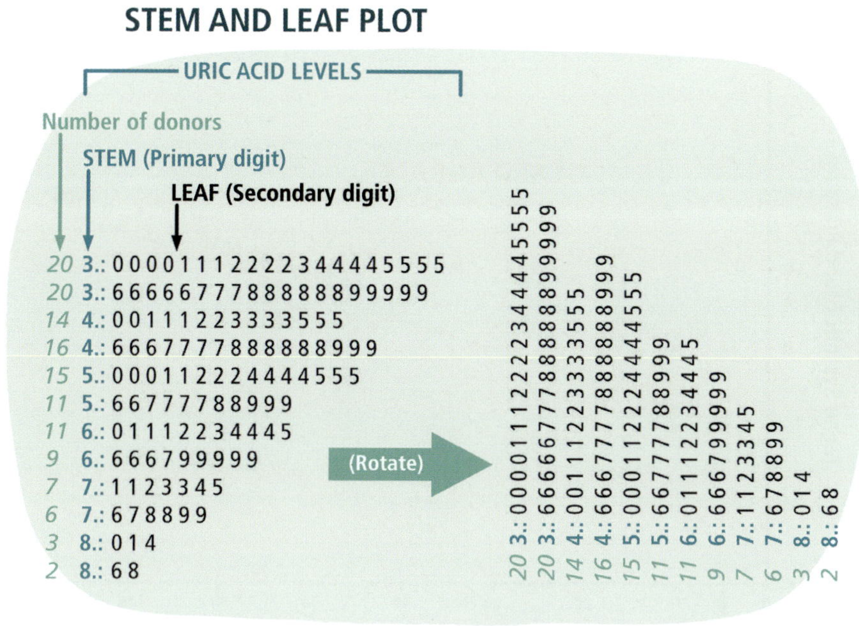

Figure 6–9. Stem-and-leaf plot.

Scattergrams

A **scattergram** is a graphical display of the data points of two variables in relation to one another. For instance, if the two variables are age and blood pressure (which increases with age), a scattergram might look something like **Fig. 6–10**, with a line of best fit drawn through the data.

Survival Curves

A **survival curve** plots survival percentage as time progresses. As **Fig. 6–11** shows, each time a patient dies, the percentage of surviving patients drops suddenly. Although the term is "survival" curve, the subject of interest doesn't necessarily have to do with patient deaths. It could, for instance, be the percentage of grafts that survive over time, the percentage of people who can hold their breath underwater as time goes by, etc.

In the case of death, for example from breast cancer, each time a patient dies, the percentage surviving decreases and is reflected as a sudden drop on the graph. There are two ways to indicate this. In the *actuarial* method, the x axis is divided into periods and after each period the changes are noted. In the *Kaplan-Meier* method, the changes are immediately noted when the patient dies. The Kaplan-Meier method is preferred, unless there are numerous patients in the study, precluding the plotting of so many points.

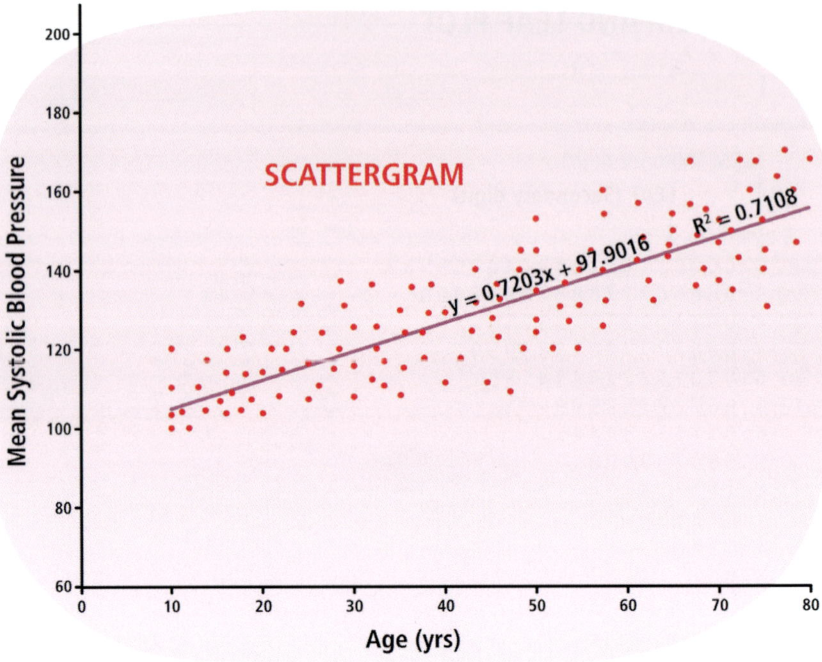

Figure 6–10. Scattergram.

There are pitfalls in survival curve graphing:

- Not every patient may enter the study at the same time. In that case, the 0 point on the x axis can be used to indicate the starting point for every patient.
- Some patients may leave the study before finishing because:

1. they moved to another town.
2. they got worse and blamed it on the treatment.
3. they got better.
4. they started a different treatment and didn't think they needed the study.
5. they suspected they were only on the placebo.

What happens to the data of patients who prematurely leave a study or otherwise do not exactly follow the protocol? Their data could be just "censored" and not used in the study (a *per protocol approach*), or it could be included, for as long as the patient was part of the study (the *intention-to-treat approach*). The researcher may work the data both ways, with and without censorship, and see if the results are similarly significant statistically. If not, there is an element of ambiguity in the study.

> *"There could be no worse experimental animals on earth than human beings: they complain, they go on vacations, they take things they are not supposed to take, they live incredibly complicated lives, and, sometimes, they do not take their medicine."*
>
> —*B. Efron*

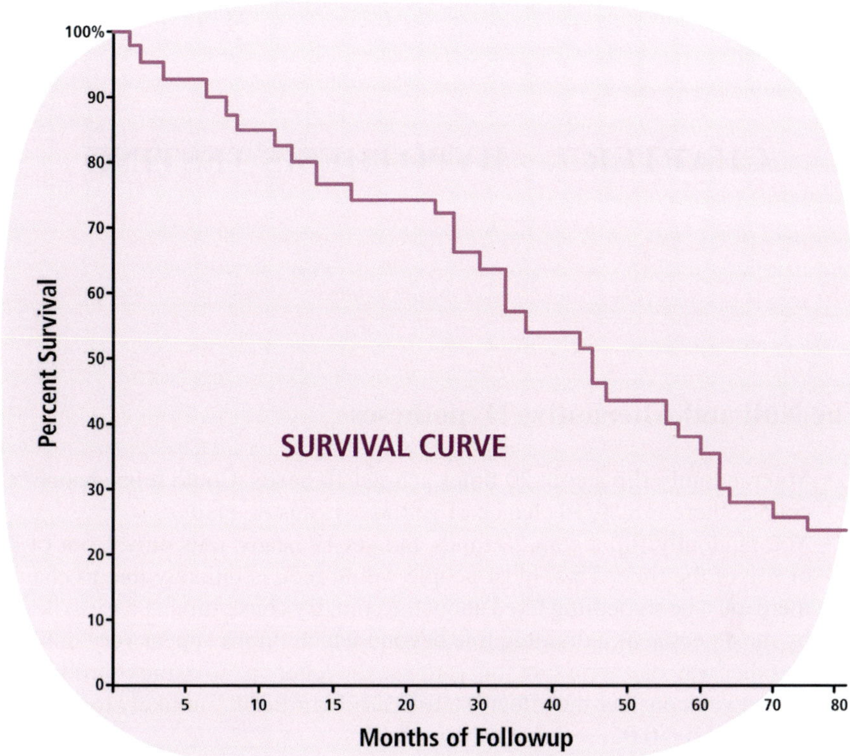

Figure 6–11. Survival curve.

Another problem: What if a new technique is developed in the course of the study that can detect breast cancer earlier? The survival curve may be prolonged simply because of the earlier detection, even though there has been no change in the actual survival time of the patient.

Question: A **pie chart** is generated to show the proportions of "yes" and "no" answers to the question, "Would you rate yourself or someone in your family as being overly concerned about germs?" The "No" slice shows 78%. The "Yes" slice shows 20%. Why don't these proportions add to 100%?

Answer: Two percent of the respondents did not answer. Always confirm that the percentages in a pie chart add up to 100%.

CHAPTER 7. HYPOTHESIS TESTING

The Null and Alternative Hypotheses

- You randomly flip a coin 20 times and get 10 heads. Could it be chance? Of course; there is a 50/50 chance of getting a heads or a tails.
- You randomly flip a coin 20 times and get 19 heads, tails only 1 out of 20, or 5% of the time. This, most people would feel, is unlikely due to chance; there must be something fixed about the coin. By convention, .05 (5%) is used by most people as a dividing line beyond which things appear very unlikely. Another way of expressing this is to use the letter "p" to express probability, so that you consider the effect "statistically significant," unlikely to be due to chance, if $p \leq 0.05$.

There is nothing magical about 5%; it's just a commonly used standard based on a subjective feeling of whether something is chance or not. If you think you are going to be sued by claiming the coin flipper is a fraud, you might want to take less risk in your assertion of trickery and establish 1% as the point where you would confidently claim the coin was fixed. This subjectively decided cutoff point is called an **alpha** value for the p (probability). It is a measure of the amount of risk you want to take in interpreting the results. It could be 1% (0.01), 5% (0.05), 10% (0.10) or any other percentage. Most of the time alpha is set at 0.05, so an experimental result that has a p-value equal to or less than 0.05 is considered statistically significant. By statistical definition, p-values that are less than or equal to 0.05 are unlikely to occur as a result of natural variation around the mean and imply that some specific situation influenced the outcome. In a research situation, the influential event is the independent variable (IV).

When alpha is set at 5%, the area under the curve in the *peripheral* 5% of the curve is termed the **critical region**. It is "critical" because values that fall outside this small area are considered statistically nonsignificant, while values inside this area are considered statistically significant.

When a p-value appears, statisticians, in their peculiar way, first employ what is termed the **null hypothesis**. For instance, if the coin flipped heads 19 times out of 20, before you've even done any math to determine probability, you first set up the null hypothesis:

1. The **null hypothesis (H_0):** The coin flips are the result of random factors and there is nothing unusual about the coin.

The **alternative hypothesis (H_1):** There is something unusual about the coin, or something besides random forces is influencing the coin.

2. Assuming you prefer to set alpha at 0.05, if the results of the flipping indicates a $p \leq 0.05$, then you *reject* the null hypothesis, since the alternative hypothesis is the more likely.

Rejecting the Null Hypothesis

Rejecting the null hypothesis does not mean the null hypothesis is incorrect, only that there is not enough evidence to support it; there might be a small chance that it is correct, or the sample size may not be large enough to feel confident that there is a significant difference. You can never disprove the null hypothesis. We can only say whether or not we have enough evidence to support the null hypothesis. *Absence of evidence is not evidence of absence.*

As a more practical example, you are trying to determine whether or not drug A has a greater effect on hypertension than drug B. The mean drop in blood pressure of drug A is found to differ from the mean drop in blood pressure of drug B. Does drug A truly have a different effect than drug B? Or could there be no difference in effect, only a seeming difference based on the random variation in the effects of drugs A and B on blood pressure? We set up two either/or hypotheses:

Null hypothesis (H_0): The mean effect of drug A on blood pressure is no different from drug B.

Alternative hypothesis (H_1) : The mean effect of drug A differs from drug B.

If the mean difference between drug A and drug B has a $p \leq .05$, we say that the result is statistically significant and reject the null hypothesis. We accept the alternative hypothesis, that the drugs most likely differ. If $p > .05$, we do not conclude that the null hypothesis is true; this doesn't mean drug A does not differ in effect from drug B, only that we do not have enough evidence to state that they do not differ. It is possible, for instance, that there were not enough people in the study to conclude for sure that there is no difference between the drugs. We could also be wrong about a conclusion that there is a statistically significant difference between the drugs; the difference could still be chance, however unlikely.

Give gold stars to research reports that use the word "estimates." This reminds readers that p-values are educated guesses.

Commonly, a scientist wishes the null hypothesis to be rejected, but sometimes may wish the opposite, e.g. if the scientist is trying to determine if a potential new drug is more harmful than the standard drug, in which case the null hypothesis is that the two drugs are equally safe, the desired hypothesis.

PART III
STATISTICAL TESTS

Parametric vs. Nonparametric Tests

The correct statistical test to use depends on the number of dependent and independent variables in the experiment, whether or not the variables are categorical or numeric, and whether the data points are Gaussian. For instance, if you test drugs A and B, and want to see their effects on blood pressure, vision, and level of drowsiness, this would involve one independent variable (the category "drugs," which has two levels, drugs A and B) and 3 dependent variables (BP, vision, and drowsiness). This will affect the choice of statistical test. Special kinds of tests are employed in epidemiology, described in **Chapter 18**.

Without getting into the math, if a frequency distribution curve of the data points has skew or kurtosis not greater than ± 2.0, it is reasonably Gaussian; it also helps to know that about half the observations are smaller than the mean; the mean and median are about the same; and that almost all the observations are within 2 standard deviations of the mean, with none more than 3 standard deviations. Parametric statistics can deal with those data. When samples are small, it is not always easy to be sure of whether or not a curve is Gaussian. In these situations, statisticians often disagree on whether to use parametric or nonparametric statistics.

Curves based on exponential changes in data may have a "**J**" shape (**Fig. 1–6**, left). It is sometimes possible to deal with such curves by transforming them so that they resemble a Gaussian curve. Skewed distributions may often be converted into a logarithmic form so that their shape resembles a normal (Gaussian) distribution (**Fig. 2–3**). Moderately skewed curves may sometimes be treated with square root transformation.

Chapters 8–16 discuss parametric tests. **Chapter 17** discusses nonparametric tests.

CHAPTER 8. DESCRIPTIVE STATISTICS

Descriptive statistics simply *describe* the data pertaining to a population or a sample, specifically the center of the data (e.g. mean, median, and mode), spread of the data points (standard deviation), and symmetry of the plotted graph.

The Z-score

Say the distribution of systolic blood pressures taken from a population of people is Gaussian and has a mean of 120 mmHg and a standard deviation of 5 mmHg. That means that about 68% of the measurements lie within 115 to 125 mmHg (5 mmHg on either side of 120) (**Fig. 8–1**). A **z-score** is the number of standard deviations that a data point (element) on a curve lies from the curve's mean:

$$z = \frac{\text{(the data point – population mean)}}{\text{population standard deviation}}$$

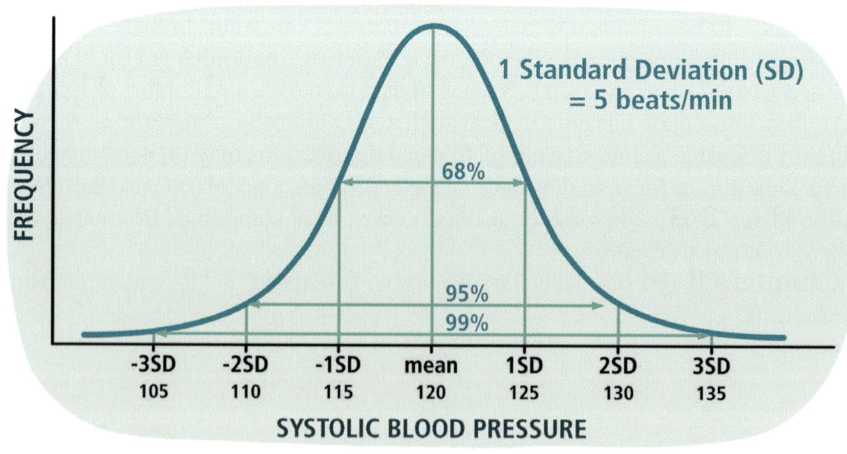

Figure 8–1. Gaussian distribution of blood pressure data.

In this case, the z-score for 125 mmHg, which is 5 mmHg (1 SD) more than the mean of 120 in **Fig. 8–1**, is (125–120)/5 = 1.

The z-score for 115 mmHg, which is 5 mmHg (1 SD) less than the mean of 120 is: (115–120)/5 = –1.

The z-score for 130 mmHg (10 mmHg more than the mean of 120) is 2: (130–120)/5 = 2.

The z-score for 110 mmHg (10 mmHg less than 120) is –2: (110–120)/5 = –2.

Z-scores cannot be used accurately on skewed populations, where the "68-95-99" rule (**Fig. 8–1**) doesn't apply.

A z-score doesn't have to be a whole number (± 1, 2, or 3). It can be any value in between, or greater than 3 or less than –3. Once you know the z-score of a single data point or sample mean, you can look it up in a z-score table (**Appendix A**) to see what percentage of the population lies at or beyond that value. For example, a z-score of 1.50 (about one and a half standard deviations; 7.5 mmHg in this case) corresponds in the table (**Appendix A**) to about .0668 (about 0.067, or 6.7%). This means that 6.7% of the people in the population have a blood pressure 127.5 mmHg [120 + (1.5 × 5) = 127.5] or higher. If the z-score were –1.50, then 6.7% of the population would have a blood pressure at or below 112.5 mmHg [120 – (1.5 × 5) = 112.5].

Once the mean and standard deviation of a Gaussian population are known, using the blood pressure case as an example, a z-score table can also be used to answer such questions as:

Question 1: What blood pressure lies at the 97.5% percentile rank of this population curve?

Answer:
Determine this as follows:

1. 2.5% of people have blood pressures at or above the 97.5th percentile.
2. Based on the z table, 0.025 (2.5%) corresponds to a z-score of about 2 (actually 1.96 if you want to be precise, using a more complete z table than in Appendix A).
3. So multiply 2 times the standard deviation of the mean (5 mmHg) and add this to the mean of 120 mmHg. That is, 120 + 2 × 5 = about 130 mmHg is the blood pressure at the 97.5th percentile of the curve.

Question 2: A person has a blood pressure of 125. The mean in the population is 120. I suspect that a blood pressure of 125 is statistically nonsignificant. Am I right?

The formal way to answer this question is through Hypothesis Testing, as follows:

First set up the null hypothesis:

Null hypothesis (H_0): This pressure of 125 is not that unusual; it's just part of the normal distribution of the population of people who have a mean BP of 120. This person with the 125 BP is simply a member of the 120 BP population.

Alternative hypothesis (H_1): This pressure of 125 is unusual; it's just too uncommon to be seriously considered as part of the normal distribution of population of people who have a mean BP of 120. This person belongs to a distinctively different population.

Answer: The population mean and its standard deviation are known to be 120 mmHg and 5 mmHg, respectively; 125 lies one standard deviation above the mean, at the 68% mark (recall the 68-95-99 rule); so 16% of people (there are 16% on either side of the inner 68% of the BPs) have blood pressures equal to or greater than 125 mmHg. This is a $p = 0.16$. This is well within statistical normality, since our chosen alpha is 0.05. We consider the results statistically nonsignificant, accept the null hypothesis and reject the alternative hypothesis. Another way of stating the data is that a blood pressure of 125 lies at the 84th percentile of the population, because 84% of the blood pressures lie below 125 (100% – 16% = 84%). (The percentile is often referred to as a *centile* (*C*), so C_{84} = 125 mmHg.)

Nowadays, a computer program will calculate the z and p-values, once the data points (elements) are put into the program.

Question 3: Lou got a test score of 550 on an exam where the school's mean is 500 and standard deviation is 100. Larry, who goes to another school, got a test score of 149 on an exam where that school's mean is 100 and standard deviation is 25. Who has the higher percentile rank?

Answer: Larry has the higher percentile rank. Why?

For Lou, $z = (550–500)/100 = 0.50$

For Larry, $z = (149–100)/25 = 1.96$

1.96 standard deviations is farther to the right of center on the curve than is 0.50. Hence, Larry is in the higher percentile. By how much? Looking at the z table:

Larry's 1.96 z-score is about 2.5% from the right side of the curve, so Larry is in the 97.50th percentile (100% − 2.5%).

Lou's 0.50 z-score is about 31% from the right side of the curve, so Lou is in about the 69th percentile. Larry's percentile is greater than Lou's by 97.5 − 69 = 28.5%.

Question 4: If the mean systolic blood pressure of the population is 120 and the standard deviation is 5, what percentage of population blood pressures lie between 115 and 125?

Answer: The 115 mmHg lies at the 16th percentile, while 125 mmHg lies at the 84th percentile. Hence, 68% of blood pressures (84% – 16% = 68%) lie between 115 and 125. By consulting a z table, you could answer the same question using other ranges, by calculating the number of SDs (the z-score) for each point and looking up each z-score in the table to determine the percentage of the curve outside that score. Then, by subtracting those percentages from one another, you can obtain the percentage of pressures that lie within that range.

CHAPTER 9. INFERENTIAL STATISTICS

Confidence Intervals vs. Hypothesis Testing and P-values

The previous chapter dealt with **descriptive statistics**; there we knew the mean and standard deviation of the population and from that we could determine where on its plotted curve a *single data point* would lie, using the z-score.

This chapter deals with **inferential statistics**. Here, we may not know the population's standard deviation or even its mean. Instead, we are presented with a sample with a particular mean and standard deviation, which we use to *infer* what that population's true mean would likely be.

For instance, say you take a random sample of 100 people in the town of Stressville, which has many thousands of people, and calculate the mean systolic blood pressure and standard deviation of this sample's mean, and it turns out this sample mean is 125, with a standard deviation of 5 mmHg. What is the true population mean in Stressville? Do the blood pressures in Stressville really differ as a whole from the rest of the USA, which has a reported population mean of 120 mmHg? Is this just a chance finding, and the difference between Stressville and the rest of the USA can be explained by natural variation in blood pressure? Or maybe there is something unusual about Stressville; maybe they all ingest too much salt, or are mutants, for instance. You want to *infer* what the mean might be in the population of Stressville. Hence "inferential" statistics.

There are two kinds of approaches to this question:

APPROACH 1: **CONFIDENCE INTERVALS (CI)**: If I took numerous samples of 100 people in Stressville, I would not expect to get a mean of 125 every time; there would be some variation. What means would I expect to get 95% of the time? This range of mean values might be, for instance, 119 to 131, and I would say "I feel 95% confident that the true population mean in Stressville lies between 119 and 131 mmHg." This range, which is now calculated by computer programs, is called a **confidence interval (CI)**. In this case, you are interested in a 95% confidence interval. (You could, for instance, be interested instead in a 90% confidence interval or a 99% confidence interval.) The values of 119 and 131 are the confidence interval **limits**. Since the 119–131 mmHg range overlaps the USA population mean of 120 mmHg, the BP in Stressville may not differ significantly from that of the USA as a whole.

Researchers, for greatest assurance of the true population mean, would like to get the smallest CI possible. CI size depends on:

1. **Sample size**. The larger the sample size, the smaller the CI, because the mean is more certain.
2. **Size of the SD**. The larger the standard deviation, the larger the CI, because the mean is less certain.
3. **Degree of confidence you want** (e.g. 95%, 90%). The higher the degree of confidence, the larger the CI. (The CI has to be larger if you want to be 99% certain that the true mean lies within it.)

APPROACH 2. **HYPOTHESIS TESTING AND P-VALUES**: Let's say the true population mean for the USA as a whole is 120. The Stressville sample is 125. What are the values that I would get 95% of the time if I repeatedly sampled the *USA population* with 100 people in each sample? A more formal way of putting this question is through the null hypothesis:

H_0: The 125 mmHg mean of the Stressville sample falls within the 95% BP range of the US population and does not represent a significantly different population.

H_1: The mean of the Stressville sample falls outside the 95% BP range of the USA population and does represent a significantly different population.

Once the calculations are done, the computer program generates a *p-value*, taking into account the sample size and the fact that you want 95% certainty (an alpha of 0.05). The p-value gives the chances that Stressville's mean of 125 falls within the 95% range around the USA average of 120. If the p-value is *greater* than 0.05, then your sample mean of 125 mmHg might by chance have come from a population whose actual mean is 120 mmHg. If $p \leq 0.05$, you likely are dealing with two different populations.

Investigators, to show significance between the Stressville and the USA population, would like to find a small p-value. The p-value depends on:

1. The difference between the means that are being compared (125 vs. 120 in this case). The larger the difference, the smaller the p-value, since it is more likely that we are dealing with two different populations.
2. The standard deviation of the sample. The larger the SD, the larger the p-value, since high variability makes the results less certain.
3. The size of the Stressville sample. The greater the Stressville sample size, the smaller the p-value, since it makes the true Stressville population more likely to be 125 mmHg.

The 95% range is exactly the same in both Approach 1 and Approach 2 (**Fig. 9–1**). It is just that in *Approach 1* (determining the 95% confidence interval), the 95% range centers around the mean of the Stressville sample.

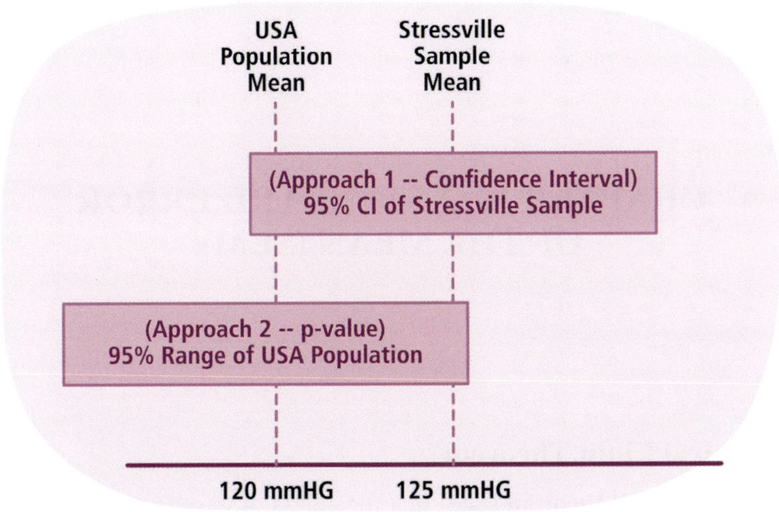

Figure 9–1. 95% confidence interval vs. 95% range in hypothesis testing with p-values.

In *Approach 2* (hypothesis testing and p-values), the 95% range centers around the mean of the USA population:

- If the 95% CI in Approach 1 (the CI approach) overlaps the mean of the USA population, the results are not statistically significant, since the mean of the USA population falls within the 95% CI range of the Stressville's mean.
- Similarly, if the range in Approach 2 (the p-value approach) overlaps Stressville's sample mean, the results are not statistically significant, since the mean of the Stressville sample would fall within the 95% range of the USA population mean. The null hypothesis is retained when the interval bars overlap the means. If the interval bars do not overlap the means, the results are statistically significant and the null hypothesis is rejected.

Do you need both a confidence interval and a p-value to assess significance? You really don't need both, but each has its advantage:

- The confidence interval gives you a meaningful range of means to look at. This range augments the information of a p-value.
- The p-value just gives you a single probability, but can be very specific about the size of the probability. Confidence intervals, though, are easier to understand and do not involve the roundabout reasoning of hypothesis testing and p-values.

How are these calculations performed? While not going into much math, it helps to mention a few points in connection with the **Central Limit Theorem** and the **Standard Error of the Mean (SEM)**.

CHAPTER 10. STANDARD ERROR OF THE MEAN (SEM)

The Central Limit Theorem

The **central limit theorem** states that regardless of the shape of a population curve, you will get a normal curve (called a **random sampling distribution of means curve**) if you take numerous repeated random samples of a set size from the population and plot the means of those samples; moreover, the mean of this plotted curve of means will be the same as the population mean.

For instance, if there is a population of 100 lottery spheres, individually labeled from 0 to 99, the curve for this distribution is a single horizontal line (**Fig. 10–1A**). However, if you repeatedly sample 2 spheres at a time from this collection and plot the means of those samples, you will get an approximately normal curve (**Fig. 10–1B**). If you took samples of 10 at a time, and plotted the means of those samples, you would also get an approximately normal curve, but one which is narrower than the 2-sample curve; samples of 50 at a time would give a still narrower curve. You would expect this, since the larger the sample, the closer you would expect the mean of each sample to be to that of the population of spheres

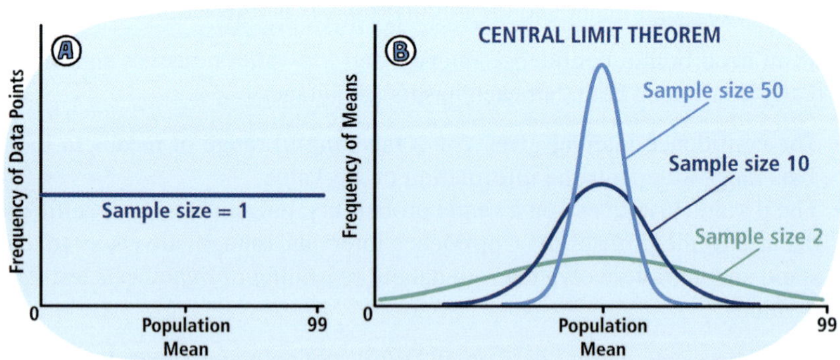

Figure 10–1. Central limit theorem. When repeatedly choosing a sphere from a cage of 99 spheres numbered from 1 to 99, the curve plots as a straight line; each sphere is picked with the same frequency as any other. With repeated samples of either 2, 10, or 50, a plot of the means follows a normal distribution, the curve becoming thinner with increased sample size.

(**Fig. 10–1B**). You would arrive at a family of curves, each member of the family representing a different sample size.

Standard Error of the Mean

The standard deviation of each of these means curves is termed a **Standard Error of the Mean** (**SEM**, sometimes written **SE**).

$$\text{SEM for a sample} = \frac{\text{Standard deviation of the sample}}{\text{Square root of the number in the sample}}$$

or

$$\text{SEM} = \text{SD}/\sqrt{\text{n}}$$

where
SD = standard deviation of the sample
n = the number of data points in the sample taken from the group

As you can see in **Fig. 10–1B** and in the equation, the larger the sample size (n), the smaller the SEM and the narrower the curve.

Just as 95% of the data in a normal curve lies within 2 standard deviations of the mean, 95% of the means in a random sampling distribution of means curve lie within 2 SEMs of the curve's mean. A 95% confidence interval for a sample thus is:

CI = the sample mean ± 2SEM

This is the general formula for calculating a confidence interval. The CI gives you an estimated range for the true population mean. You can be 95% sure that the true population mean lies within the 95% confidence interval. In other words, the true population mean would lie within the CI in 95% of the samples.

Confidence intervals are frequently used in surveys. For instance "the survey showed 60% of people ± 3% prefer brand A over brand B." The 3% (2 SEMs) reflects a sample size of about 1000 people, which is common in surveys and polls.

For a reasonably large sample (30 or more elements), the sample mean plus or minus one SEM is a confidence interval of 68%. Plus or minus two SEMs (1.96 precisely) represent a confidence interval of 95% (the most commonly used in research); plus or minus 3 (2.58 precisely) SEMs represent a 99% confidence interval.

Standard deviation and SEM are both described in the same measuring units. However, SEM, unlike a standard deviation, is *not* a measure of spread of the data in the sample or population. Rather, it is a measure of how well you know the population mean. While a standard deviation may not change much when changing sample size, an SEM gets smaller the larger the sample size. With an enormous sample size, SEM reduces to close to zero, since, with very large samples, there is little doubt as to the mean of the true population. If the sample size were infinite, the SEM would be zero and the CI would simply be the sample mean, the same as the population mean, since the sample then *is* the population. An SEM can be very small even if the standard deviation is large, if the sample size is very large. The SEM is always smaller than the standard deviation. A small SEM suggests that the sample mean is close to the population mean.

The SEM is reported in the literature as a way to show how well you know the population mean. Psychologically, since the SEM is smaller than the SD, it can give the reader the false impression that the scatter of data points is small, when this is not the case. Just reporting the sample mean and standard deviation, however, doesn't give you any idea of how well you know the population mean, because the sample mean and SD refer only to a sample of data. Even better than reporting the SEM, though, is reporting the confidence interval, which gives you a good idea of the likely range for the population mean.

As mentioned, the 95% confidence interval for a sample is:

CI = the sample mean ± 2SEM

There is a caveat to this description, which depends on sample size:

When the sample sizes are small (less than about 30), the "2" in the CI formula has to be modified somewhat to allow for sample size through what is called a **t table** (**Appendix B**). When you go to a t table, you first select the sample size. In the table, sample size is indicated by **degrees of freedom (df)**, which for our purposes is just the number of elements in the sample minus one (n–1). For instance, if your sample size is 10, the degrees of freedom (df) is 9.

You also have to select the column that indicates that you are looking for a 95% CI, which is almost always the case, rather than some other percentage; t tables usually list other percentage levels as well (such as 90% or 99%). For a 95% CI, you would look for the value of t under an alpha of $p = 0.05$. The t table in **Appendix B** is simplified to only include values for a 95% CI.

The t-value in the table (look at the "two-tailed" column; the "one-tailed" column will be explained shortly in the "One vs. Two-Tailed Studies" **in Chapter 12**) is then substituted for the "2" in the CI equation for greater accuracy. Most t-values (those of sample sizes of 30 or more) are close to 2 (for two-tailed tests), but not exactly. The more exact equation then becomes:

CI = the sample mean ± t* SEM

The t* in this equation is the t-value you get from a t table for the specific row that indicates degrees of freedom.

CHAPTER 11. THE t-TEST

The Meaning of the t-Test

Unlike the calculation of a confidence interval, in which your sample mean is not being compared with any other mean, you do compare two means in hypothesis testing with a t-test.

For instance, when you find that your sample mean in Stressville is 125 mmHg and you want to know with 95% certainty what the true population mean is for Stressville, you present a *confidence interval* for this. In *hypothesis testing*, though, you may want to compare the Stressville sample mean of 125 with a proposed general population mean of 120, to determine whether or not the two means are really part of the same population. To do this, you need to calculate a t-value of the difference between these means, namely:

$$t = \frac{\text{(Sample mean – population mean)}}{\text{Sample SEM}}$$

which in this case would be:

t = (125–120)/Sample SEM

The calculation of a t-value is comparable to a z-score mentioned in Chapter 8:

$$z = \frac{\text{(the data point – population mean)}}{\text{population standard deviation}}$$

That calculated t-value is compared with the t* value in the t table. If the calculated t-value is equal or greater than the table t*-value, the results are statistically significant. If it is less than the table t*-value, then the results are statistically nonsignificant. This is called doing a **t-test**. The t-value in the t table indicates the number of SEMs that would be needed to establish statistical significance. This t-value in the table is the **critical value** for statistical significance.

Comparing Two Samples

A **z-score** is used to compare *one data point* with a known population whose mean and standard deviation are known. A **z-test** is used to compare a *sample* *mean* with a known population whose mean and standard deviation are known, as follows: Note that the formula above for calculating the z-score of a data point requires knowledge of the population standard deviation. So does the formula for calculating the z-score of a sample mean, which is:

$$z = \frac{\text{(the sample mean – population mean)}}{\text{population SEM}}$$

But knowing the SEM of the population requires knowing the population's SD, which is almost always unknown. Therefore, a **t-test** is used when the population SD is not known.

A **single sample t-test** compares a sample mean to a known population mean (like comparing the Stressville sample mean with the mean of the USA population).

An **independent samples (unpaired) t-test** compares two distinct samples (like comparing Stressville's sample with a sample from neighboring Worrytown). Here we are not sure of the population mean of either sample. As a common example, is the effect of a new, and highly expensive, drug A any better than the effect of old, reliable and inexpensive drug B?

A **dependent samples (paired) t-test** compares two *matched* samples (like comparing the Stressville sample with the same Stressville people the previous year). Sample sizes need to be equal for a paired t-test. Paired t-tests, since they use matching samples, are less susceptible to selection error than are independent t-tests, since you are matching a group with itself. Therefore, cultural background, heredity, environmental exposure, gender, and many other variables are less likely to differ with the before-and-after picture as compared with two different groups of people, where assorted variables can throw off the accuracy of the calculations. This situation entails a mathematical modification to the t-test, which will not be discussed here.

Different kinds of situations allow paired t-tests. For instance:

1. Comparing the before and after of a treatment on a single patient.
2. Comparing treatment on one side of the body with the other in a single patient.
3. Comparing one twin with the other.
4. Close matching of two different groups for many variables, such as age, gender, cultural and economic background, medical history, education, and area of residence.

The subject of the central limit theorem and SEMs can be difficult to fully understand without a deeper understanding of the underlying math, which is beyond the scope of this book. In case your reaction is like that of SEM Sam in **Fig. 11–1**, not to worry. There is a bottom line. That is to just look at the calculated confidence interval and p-value in the research report. That will give you a relatively good idea of the likely range for the population mean and statistical significance of the results. If the SEM is reported, it is an estimation of how well

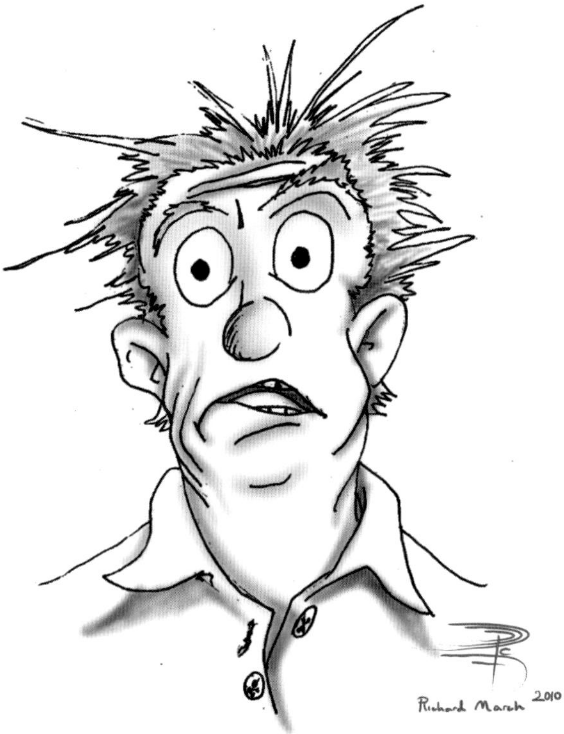

Figure 11–1. SEM Sam. Stunned reaction on not fully understanding the meaning of Standard Error of the Mean (SEM).

you know the true population mean. For a small SEM (which is desired), the smaller the confidence interval and more certain the population mean. For a large SEM, the wider the confidence interval and the less certain the population mean. However, the confidence interval alone is intuitively easier to comprehend than the SEM.

CHAPTER 12. ONE-TAILED VS. TWO-TAILED STUDIES

The Two-Tailed Test

In doing a t-test you declare, in advance of an experiment, that you will use an alpha of 0.05 (or some other value) to determine significance. You must *also* declare whether this alpha you talk about is **one-tailed** or **two-tailed**. As **Fig. 12–1A** shows, 95% of the data lie in the center of the curve; 5% lie in the periphery: 2.5% on the right and 2.5% on the left. These 2.5% regions are termed **critical regions**. If the results fall outside these critical 2.5% regions, within the 95% probability area, the p is then > 0.05 and you cannot call the results significant. *This is a two-tailed (nondirectional) setup.*

As a specific example, you may want to compare the mean effect of a new experimental drug with the mean effect of a placebo on reduction of cardiac arrhythmias. You may not know before the study whether the drug will show an improvement over the placebo and result in a significant decrease in cardiac arrhythmias, or whether it may actually be more harmful, causing worsening of the arrhythmias. You announce in advance a two-tailed study with an alpha of 0.05. Since you are allowing for the possibilities that the drug may be either harmful or helpful, then the 5% you have allotted to probability is split between the right and left ends of the curve. The cutoff point between statistically likely is 0.025 on the right and 0.025 on the left, totaling 0.05, *two* critical regions.

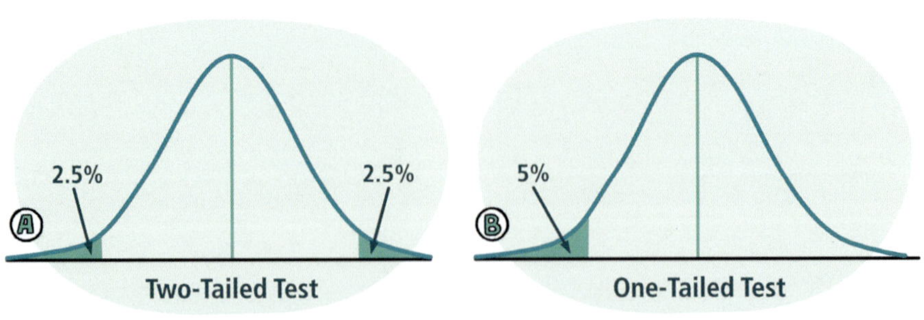

Figure 12–1. Two-tailed vs. one-tailed tests. In this case, the alpha is 0.05 for both tests, but is split in the two-tailed test.

If the results fall within either of these two critical .025 regions in this two-tailed study, the results are considered statistically significant for either improvement or failure, depending on which side of the curve the results fall. If the results fall outside the critical regions (are in the central region of the curve), you will end up with a statistically nonsignificant result. If the results fall within the right-hand critical region, indicating that administration of the drug has been accompanied by an increase in (worsening of) arrhythmias, you declare that the results are statistically significant for worsening. If the results fall within the left-hand critical region, indicating that administration of the drug has been accompanied by improvement in (lessening of) arrhythmias, you declare that the results are statistically significant for improvement.

The One-Tailed Test

In the arrhythmia case, though, let's say that this was a two-tailed test, and what actually happened was that the results fell just outside the left-hand critical region, not quite significant for arrhythmia improvement. You really want to see arrhythmia improvement and are disappointed in the less-than-significant results. In retrospect, if you had thought for sure that the drug was going to be helpful, you may have wanted, in planning the experiment, to bet all your 5% alpha on the left side of the curve, **as in Fig. 12-1B.** Both curves A and B have an alpha of 0.05, but the two-tailed test splits alpha into two 0.025 areas, while the one-tailed test bets the entire alpha on one large 0.05 tail, the critical region for the one-tailed test. The 5% proportion of data in the one-tailed test can either be the left (lower) tail or the right (upper) tail, but not both.

Then, if you posed a one-tailed hypothesis, did the same experiment and came up with the same data for arrhythmia improvement as the two-tailed test the results would fall within that 5% critical region of the left-hand side of the curve. This would be statistically significant, and you would happily report that the results are significant for improvement with the drug.

Unfortunately, it is tempting for a researcher who has announced a two-tailed test (most studies are two-tailed) and finds a p-value indicating non-significance to change the setup to a one-tailed test as an afterthought, in which case the p-value will typically be about half, about 0.03 in this case. *But you can't just change your hypothesis after the fact.* This is an example of "P-ing (Pee-ing) all over the place," discussed in the next chapter. You have to announce in advance whether your study is going to be one-tailed or two-tailed. Some journals will only accept a two-tailed experiment, out of concern that the investigator had a change of mind after the experiment and changed the experiment to a one-tailed one.

In addition, if you announced in advance that the experiment would be one-tailed, betting all 5% on improvement, but the results unexpectedly indicated clearly that the drug was harmful, you cannot ethically just switch to a two-tailed test and announce that the drug is harmful. It's too late. All you can say is that the study did not yield significant results. You will have to repeat the experiment to confirm that the drug is harmful. (See "P-ing all over the place" in Chapter 13.)

The statistical software may ask whether you wish to do a one or two-tailed test and take that into consideration in the calculations. If it only provides a two-tailed p-value, use half of the p-value that it generates if you intend that the study be one-tailed.

For a *single sample t-test*, results would look something like this, for a study, say, where you were trying to determine whether or not medical students used more or less aspirin than the general population:

"There was a significant difference between medical student annual aspirin use (two-tailed test; M = 113 aspirin/yr; SD = 13.04), and the national average (μ = 130 aspirin/yr, t(4) = –2.92, p = 0.04)."

M stands for the mean medical student aspirin use; μ stands for mean general population use. The "4" in parenthesis refers to degrees of freedom. There were 5 students in the study. The "t" of –2.92 is the calculated value of t. The t table value for t, where df = 4 for a two-tailed t-test looking for 95% certainty is –2.776. Since –2.92 (the minus sign indicates that the t-value is on the left side of the curve) extends beyond –2.776 into the critical zone, this indicates statistical significance for students taking fewer aspirins.

The CI part of the report might read:

"The 95% CI is –33.19, –.8107," showing that medical students average somewhere between 1–33 fewer aspirin than the rest of the population. The fact that the CI numbers do not cross 0 indicates statistical significance, since 95% of the time, students would be taking fewer aspirin than the general population (the difference between the students and the general population is not zero).

The report style looks similar for independent samples t-tests and paired samples t-tests, although the formulas for the calculations (today done by computer) are somewhat different.

For an *unpaired t-test* (*independent t-test*) that studied whether a sample of men consumed more or less aspirin than a sample of women, results might read:

"An unpaired t-test was performed. There was a significant effect of gender on mean annual aspirin consumption, t(10) = –3.11, p = 0.011, in which women took more aspirin than men." The degrees of freedom here is a combination of two groups [6 men and 6 women; df = (6–1) + (6–1) = 10].

For a *paired t-test*, trying to determine whether or not a sample of patients took more aspirin when they had a sprained ankle, results might read something like:

"Patients reported no differences in aspirin use in the presence and absence of a sprained ankle, t(4) = 1.53, p = 0.20."

The sign of the t-value indicates the location of the t-value, the right tail for positive t-values and the left for negative t-values.

Doing a **t-test** requires input of:

1. the desired alpha value
2. indication of whether this is a one-tailed or two-tailed study

3. indication of whether this is a single-sample, paired, or an unpaired t-test
4. the known means and standard deviations of the population (if known) and sample(s)

The computer will then do the necessary calculations and provide you with a confidence interval and p-value.

Different mathematical approaches are used for single sample, independent, and paired t-tests. The math can get complicated here, but bypassing the math, the computer calculations for all these t-tests result in a t-value, confidence interval, and a p-value. A study may report the t-value, degrees of freedom, confidence interval, SEM, standard deviation, p-value, and whether the test is one-tailed or two-tailed.

CHAPTER 13. P-ING (PEE-ING) ALL OVER THE PLACE

I look at the serial number of a dollar that I have removed from my wallet. I announce that the serial number is G87181338D. There are billions of dollar bills in circulation. What are the chances that I would have this particular serial number on my dollar bill? One in billions. Are you impressed? Are you ready to declare a miracle?

No, because I looked in advance.

Nor would I fool anyone if I didn't look in advance, but simply said, after the fact, that this was the serial number I had in mind. Oh yeah.

Nor would I be fooling anyone if I had a list of the serial numbers of all dollar bills in the USA and announced that the one in your wallet was one of them. Of course it would be one of them, since the list consists of the serial numbers of all dollar bills.

On the other hand, if I never had that list, and never looked at the dollar bill, and declared that the one I was going to pull out of your wallet had that serial number, this would be an amazing coincidence; I would be the celebrity of the paranormal world. The degree of amazement depends on whether or not I had this prior information.

Similarly, whether or not to accept that a p-value is significant depends on whether you have declared your hypothesis in advance of the study, and also on how many hypotheses you are testing. For instance, if I say that the drug Dammitol will lower blood pressure, and unexpectedly find that there was a higher percentage of people who benefited from the drug who also were born under the astrological sign of Sagittarius, and the p-value for this coincidence occurring was < 0.05, do I get excited and hypothesize that people born under Sagittarius will have a better effect with this drug, and do I report this in the *Journal of Parapsychological Phenomena*, if not the *New England Journal of Medicine*? Of course not (well, maybe the parapsychological journal). Saying "$p = 0.05$" simply means that you will get the same result on the basis of random sampling 1 out of 20 times. There are hundreds of unlikely correlations that may occur in an experiment. If one of them pops up with a p of 0.05 or less (a Sagittarius relationship), that would be expected, given so many potential hypotheses. If you announced the Sagittarius hypothesis before doing the study, then it would be more impressive than finding a Sagittarius connection after the experiment is done. If you announced the Sagittarius hypothesis after the study, that would be "P-ing all over the place."

> *"If the fishing expedition catches a boot, the fishermen should throw it back, not claim that they were fishing for boots."*
>
> —J.L. Mills

This does not mean that the boot that you caught (an unplanned hypothesis that turned out to be significant) is useless. You may have come across something important, but your results are spoiled. You have to repeat the experiment to see if you can duplicate the results.

It is important not only to announce in advance of the experiment what hypothesis you are advancing, but also how many hypotheses you want to advance. The more hypotheses, the greater the chance that at least one of them will turn out with a p of 0.05 or less by chance alone, even if they are all individually highly improbable.

The **Bonferroni method** is a simple way to deal with multiple hypotheses. If the number of proposed hypotheses is 5, for instance, divide your alpha of 0.05 by 5, giving a new target alpha of 0.01. You will then have to show that level of significance for each comparison to be able to declare that your results are statistically significant. The Bonferroni method loses accuracy after about 10 hypotheses, so other, more complex, statistical methods can be used when dealing with multiple hypotheses, but these are beyond the scope of this book.

CHAPTER 14. TYPE I AND TYPE II ERRORS

Type I and Type II Errors

Say you set alpha at p = 0.05 and you get the result p = 0.03. You declare that you have gotten a positive result, namely the result is statistically significant, and you reject the null hypothesis. But what if you are wrong and this positive result is just a chance finding? You have then committed what is termed a **Type I error**, a **false positive**.

Conversely, if your p comes out 0.07, you declare that the results are not statistically significant and you retain the null. But what if you are wrong and the alternative hypothesis is really correct? You have then committed a **Type II error**, a **false negative**.

Mnemonic: You can remember that Type I is false Positive, because both the "I" in "Type I" and the "P" in "false Positive" contain a single vertical line. You can remember that Type II is false Negative, because both the "II" in Type II and the "N" in "false Negative" contain 2 vertical lines.

When alpha is set very low, e.g., 0.01 instead of 0.05, this reduces the chance of committing a Type I error (getting a false positive) since the chances of getting a significant result by chance would have to be equal or less than 1 in a hundred. Reducing the chance of a Type I error, however, increases the chance of a Type II error. Similarly, increasing the alpha from 0.05 to 0.10 reduces the chance of committing a Type II error, but increases the chance of a Type I error. The only way to simultaneously reduce the chance of both types of error is to increase the sample size, which increases certainty all around.

The value of alpha is a measure of the risk you're willing to take in interpreting the results. For instance, if your experiment explores your hypothesis that a very expensive and toxic drug cures cancer, you set up a null hypothesis:

H_0 (null hypothesis): Drug and placebo are equally effective.
H_1 (alternative hypothesis): The drug is more effective than placebo.

If you set the alpha at 0.05 and your results indicate a p = 0.04, you would conclude that the results are significant and the drug is likely better than a placebo. But the drug is toxic and expensive, and there is always a chance that you are wrong, a

Type I (false positive) error, in which case you would be prescribing a toxic, expensive drug that is no better than placebo. You may want to set the alpha lower, say 0.01, at the outset of the study to be more certain that the drug is really effective.

On the other hand, say you test an inexpensive new drug that has no side effects for its ability to cure cancer. You set up the same null hypothesis:

H_0: Drug and placebo are equally effective.
H_1: The drug is more effective than placebo.

Then if you set alpha at 0.05 and you get a p = 0.07, the experiment lacks statistical significance; do you tell doctors not to use the drug, because there is no evidence that it works? What if you are wrong, and the drug really cures cancer, a Type II (false negative) error? You would be missing the opportunity to provide cancer patients with a viable therapeutic agent. You might want, in advance of the study, to set alpha at 0.10; that would make 0.07 statistically significant and you would declare that the drug holds promise in the treatment of cancer. What would you have to lose? If the drug turns out to be just a placebo, this would not be as bad a mistake as missing the opportunity to use an effective, inexpensive, nontoxic cancer drug. Setting the alpha value is a subjective decision that depends on the risk you are willing to take in interpreting the results, but alpha is commonly set at a p = 0.05.

Power

The chance of committing a Type I error is equal to the alpha value. If alpha, for instance, is 0.01, then if you find a p = 0.01, the chance that the result could happen by chance (rather than the independent variable) is 1 in 100 times. The chance of committing a Type II error is called **beta**. It is not that forthright to calculate beta, and the math will not be presented here, but is important to know something about **power**:

Power = (1 – beta). Power is the likelihood that if the results are found statistically nonsignificant, then the relationship you are studying *really is* nonsignificant and you have not committed a Type II error. Let's look at this with an analogy:

Say there is a dark cave and you send in someone to determine whether or not the cave is empty. The person comes out and says it's empty. Is the person correct? It's dark in the cave, so maybe he made a mistake; you're not sure. However, if he goes in with a flashlight, the power from the flashlight will illuminate the cave. Then, when he comes out and says it's empty, you have greater confidence that his negative report is correct. The greater the power of a test, the more assured one can be that the negative result that is reported is really true. You would like a test to have high power.

Most researchers set ideal power at about 0.80, although others, who want to be even more certain that the negative result is correct, may be more stringent and set the ideal power higher, such as 0.95. The problem with just increasing the power, though, is that while it reduces the chance of a Type II error, it increases the chance of a Type I error.

Decreasing alpha reduces the chance of a Type I error but decreases power and increases the chance of a Type II error. The way to simultaneously reduce the chances of both a Type I and Type II error is to increase the sample size.

Power is increased when:

1. sample size is increased
2. standard deviations are small
3. effect size (described below) is increased

Effect Size

When the effect of a drug is compared with placebo, you may get a p of 0.05 or less, indicating that the drug effect is significantly different from placebo. However, statistically significant does not necessarily mean clinically significant. For instance, a weight loss drug may reduce a person's weight over 2 months by one ounce as compared with a placebo, and this difference may be found to be significantly different from placebo if the sample size is large enough. However, no one would be impressed with this result; it is not *clinically* significant even though it is *statistically* significant. One way to convey the degree of clinical significance to the reader is simply to say how much weight was lost. The reader sees "one ounce more than a placebo" over two months and rightfully is not going to be impressed.

However, what if the mean weight loss on the drug was 22 lbs as compared with the placebo, where the mean weight loss was 2 lbs? Surely, that would subjectively satisfy a person that the regimen was effective; simply subtract 22 – 2 = a 20 lb difference between treatment and control; very nice, presumably.

The problem with this approach, though, is that while you like the idea of the loss of 20 lbs, which is the difference between the means of the treatment and control, you need to know the variation among persons taking the regimen and placebo. For instance, some people in the placebo group may have also lost 22 lbs, others nothing, or gained weight, giving a mean weight loss of the control of 2 lbs. There may similarly be variation in the treatment group. If there is a lot of variability within each group, the difference between groups is less impressive; some of the difference may be due to random variation. To what degree can we attribute the effect to a true difference between treatment and control as opposed to random variation? You have to take into account the variation (standard deviation) within each group.

One way (**Cohen's d**) is to subtract the means of the two groups from one another and divide by the standard deviation, assuming the SD of each group is the same.

$$\text{Cohen's d} = \frac{(\text{Mean1} - \text{Mean2})}{\text{SD}}$$

Cohen suggested that an effect size of 0.2, calculated through his formula, is a *small* effect, 0.5 *medium* and 0.8 or higher *large*, to help you decide whether or not the results are really impressive. The research paper might read something like:

> "There was a significant effect of gender on mean annual aspirin consumption, $t(10) = -3.11$, $p = 0.011$. The effect of gender was large, Cohen's $d = 1.82$."

When the SDs of the groups differ, one way to find effect size is to only use the SD of the control group (**Glass's delta**) in the calculation. There are other more complex ways to calculate effect, taking into account not only the SDs of both groups, but also the size of the samples. This would be a good place to say that these methods are beyond the scope of this book.

The power of a test is increased when the effect size is increased, whether by increased difference between the means or by decreased standard deviation (as per the Cohen's d formula above).

Question: Lab #1 and Lab #2 independently compare the effectiveness of drug A with that of drug B. Lab #1 uses 250 subjects and arrives at a $p < 0.05$, which suggests there is a significant different between the drugs. Lab #2 uses only 25 subjects and arrives at a $p > 0.05$, which suggests that any differences are nonsignificant. Which lab is more likely to be correct? On the one hand, the inclination might be to choose Lab #1 because of its large number of subjects. However, the t-value in the t table takes into account the smaller sample size. So are the two studies equally credible?

Answer: The smaller study is less credible since there is a greater chance of sampling error. Also, smaller studies have less power and an increased chance for a Type II (false negative) error. Any analysis using t-tests in which there are fewer than 30 individuals in each group is generally not trustworthy.

Bayesian Thinking

In **Bayesian thinking**, the researcher combines the statistical results of the experiment with previous knowledge to help determine whether or not the results are really significant. While this can be a complex mathematical consideration that is beyond the scope of this book, there is also an intuitive approach to Bayesian thinking.

For instance, if the study generates a p of 0.06, the immediate impulse may be to declare the result statistically nonsignificant, and that is the end of the matter. However, in Bayesian thinking, the researcher may know that previous results and knowledge point to a significant relationship, and this previous information influences judgment toward thinking that the 0.06 should not be dismissed so readily; there may well be a significant relationship. The meaning of the p-value relates to its context.

Similarly, if the result is a p of 0.04, this should not necessarily lead the investigator to proclaim statistical significance. The whole idea of such a statistically significant relationship may not make sense physiologically, and conflict greatly with previous knowledge. So the researcher is more willing to consider that 0.04 may have been a statistical fluke.

On the other hand if the p is 0.00001, then despite previous knowledge to the contrary, the researcher needs to seriously consider that there is a real statistical significance here. As Sherlock Holmes stated, *"When you have eliminated the impossible, whatever remains, however improbable, must be the truth."*

Calculation of Sample Size

Don't change the sample size after the experiment! If the result is barely significant statistically, the researcher may feel that if only he had a larger sample size in the study, he could get that p under 0.05, so he continues the experiment, adding more people. That is a no-no, because the research then is not aimed for the truth, but rather at forcefully arriving at a desired p-value, stopping when the p reaches 0.05 or less. Had he continued beyond that point, perhaps the results would be even less significant than originally, but he won't allow this to happen; the researcher wants to stop when the data fits his preconceived notions. That is dishonest. That is why it is important, before the study is done, to calculate the estimated sample size needed for the study. But how do you do that?

The equations for determining the p-value of a relationship between two groups take into account the means of the two groups, the standard deviations of the groups, and the number of elements in each group. Once these are plugged into the equation, a p-value comes out and if you are interested in being 95% sure of the results, you can note if this p-value is 0.05 or less.

The same equations for power and calculating t-values can be used to calculate desired sample size, only instead of calculating what the p-value is, you put the desired 0.05 p-value into the equation and then solve the equation for sample size (n). The result will give you an estimated sample size necessary to arrive at a p-value of 0.05. The calculation process is not actually that simple and requires a knowledgeable statistician, who may use a computer program to do the calculations. Determining sample size involves the following considerations:

1. What is the smallest effect that would be of clinical importance? It requires a larger sample size to detect a small effect.
2. Are you going to use a surrogate endpoint (e.g. CD4+ count rather than deaths from HIV)? This will influence sample size.
3. What power do you want? Plug that into the power equation to determine sample size.
4. What alpha do you want?
5. What confidence interval do you want (e.g. 95%, 99% etc)? Knowing that, you can calculate sample size for that CI. In view of the equation $SEM = SD/\sqrt{n}$, note that in order to halve a confidence interval, the sample size has to be increased by a factor of 4. This could require a very large sample.
6. Which statistical test will you use?
7. Will you use a one-tailed or a two-tailed t-test?
8. How many patient dropouts do you expect?

9. How uncommon is the disease? If the disease is rare, you may need a larger sample to determine whether a preventative, such as a new vaccine, will work.
10. How big are the groups' standard deviations (if known)? A larger sample size is needed the larger the groups' standard deviations.

Once you have decided on a sample size, it is best to plan for an even larger sample size to allow for subjects who may drop out of the study.

Researchers often don't plan optimal sample size before doing the experiment. Then they find that they are short on numbers and repeat the experiment with still more numbers. This spoils the interpretation of the results, since the research will simply stop when the researcher gets the results he wants.

"To call in the statistician after the experiment is done may be no more than asking him to perform a post-mortem examination: he may be able to say what the experiment died of."

—R. Fisher

CHAPTER 15. ANOVA (ANALYSIS OF VARIANCE)

ANOVA and F-ratio

A t-test is used when you want to compare the sample means of two groups. For instance, "Does the degree of pain relief from morphine differ from that of hydromorphone?"

When there are 3 or more groups (for instance a comparison of morphine, hydromorphone, and placebo), you could use multiple t-tests, comparing morphine with hydromorphone; morphine with placebo; and hydromorphone with placebo. However, not only can this consume time when there are many groups, but the use of multiple t-tests makes the study unreliable, for statistical significance may then occur simply because multiple hypotheses are being tested, the "p-ing all over the place problem," with a resulting Type I (false positive) error. ANOVA avoids this problem by looking at all the groups at once.

ANOVA asks "Is there some relationship that is statistically significant when considering all the groups as a whole?" An **F-ratio** is used to determine this. The F-ratio calculation depends on two questions:

1. What is the variability *between* the groups?
2. What is the variability *within* each group?

$$F = \frac{\text{(variance } \textit{between} \text{ the groups)}}{\text{(variance } \textit{within} \text{ each group)}}$$

Rather than go into the mathematics, think intuitively of "variance" as being "variability." The greater the variability *between* the groups as opposed to the variability *within* each group, the higher the F ratio. The F ratio will be near 1 if there is no significant difference between the groups.

A computer program calculates a p-value from the F ratio. Research reports commonly list the results of the division of the F ratio as the **F statistic**, in addition to the p-value and confidence interval. If F is large, p will be small. (Similarly, in the t-test, when t is large, p will be small.)

The ANOVA test can be phrased using the null hypothesis:

Null Hypothesis (H_0): The means of all the groups are equal, and any differences are due to random forces (chance).

Alternative Hypothesis (H_1): Not all the group means are equal. At least one of the groups differs from the rest.

If the alternative hypothesis is true, the F statistic alone does not tell us which group, or groups, are responsible for the statistically significant variability. Additional calculations can tell us that and point to how the factors of each group interact with one another. **Fig. 15–1** illustrates this intuitively.

Both ANOVA and t-tests assume not only that samples were drawn randomly, but also that the populations from which samples are drawn have the same variance. **Levene's test** is often used to see if variances in the compared samples differ significantly or not. This time, you do not want a significant difference. If Levene's p-value is less than 0.05, the variances are not homogeneous. This must

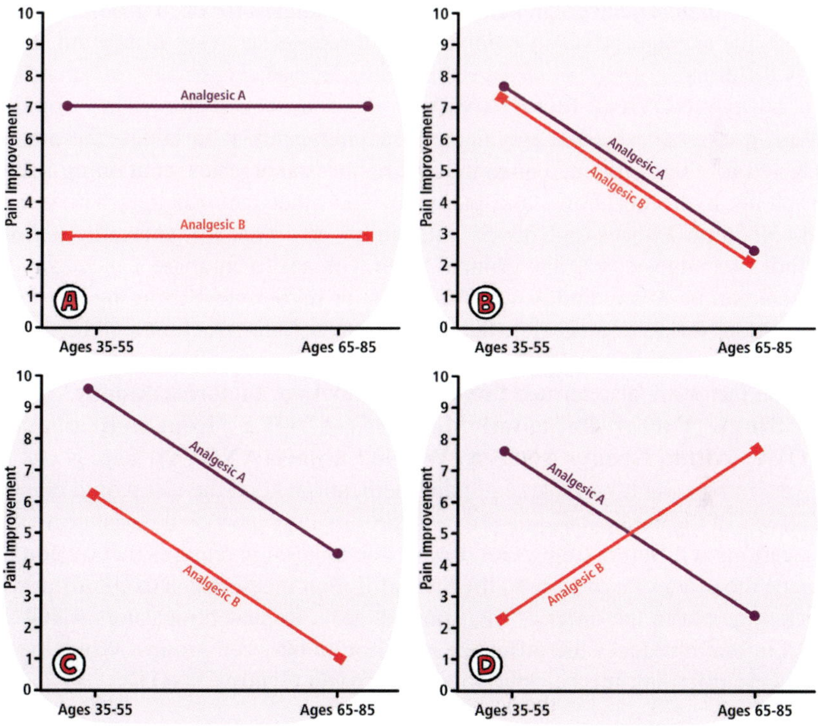

Figure 15–1. Relation of variables in an ANOVA test, visualized intuitively. This study compares pain improvement with analgesics A and B in two age groups. The analgesic and age groups are independent variables. Pain relief is the dependent variable.

- In the relationships of **Fig. 15–1A**, ANOVA shows the *main effect* on pain is due to the drugs, not to age.
- In **Fig. 15–1B**, the main effect is due to age, not to the drugs.
- In **Fig. 15–1C**, there are two main effects on pain, that due to the drugs, and that due to age.
- In **Fig. 15–1D**, the lines cross, termed an **interaction**. Unlike **Figs 15–1A**, **B**, and **C**, where the lines are parallel, there is no simple one-on-one relationship between drugs and pain, or age and pain. The relationships are more complex and have to be examined more closely.

be dealt with (e.g. transforming the data, beyond the scope of this book) before doing statistical tests to compare means.

The concept of one- and two-tailed tests, which applies to t-tests, does not apply to ANOVA tests.

In **1-way ANOVA** (also called **1-factor ANOVA**), only one independent variable **factor** is examined. A single factor, for instance, could be drugs for pain (analgesics). Morphine, hydromorphone, and placebo are each **levels** (versions) of the factor. Thus, the single factor (independent variable) of analgesics contains in this study 3 levels: morphine, hydromorphone, and placebo.

The patients might be divided into 3 groups of 15 patients, one group taking morphine, the second group hydromorphone, and the third group placebo. This arrangement, where each patient receives only one level of the factor is termed **between groups design**. Patients would rate their pain, say, 30 minutes after taking their medication using a 10-point scale where 0 = no pain and 10 = worst imaginable pain. The average pain would be calculated for each group, using the mean as the average. ANOVA compares the three means to see if they are significantly different.

In **2-way ANOVA (2-factor ANOVA)**, there are two factors. They could be, for instance, analgesics and age, namely two independent variables (factors) that are tested for their influence on pain. One factor is analgesics, containing 3 levels (morphine, hydromorphone, and placebo). The other factor is age, which might be divided into 2 levels (age 35–55 and age 65–85). That would require 6 groups (3 kinds of analgesics × 2 age groups), with 6 means to compare.

There can be 3-way and 4-way ANOVAs, or higher, depending on how many independent variable categories (factors) there are. A third factor could be sex, and a fourth factor could be cultural background, for instance. ANOVAs with more than one factor are also termed **factorial ANOVAs** or **factorial designs**.

In **Single Factor Repeated Measures ANOVA (Repeated measures ANOVA; Within Groups ANOVA; Within Subjects ANOVA)**, there is one factor (one independent variable, e.g. pain medications) and the test would compare the effects of the medications on only *one* group of people who have taken all three medications at different times. Good experimental design requires that we counterbalance the order of exposure to the three different medications to control for any effects inherent in the order of their presentation. Repeated measures ANOVA is useful in that it reduces the influence of variation between groups. When the two groups are different, it is referred to as a **Between Groups ANOVA**.

MANOVA and ANCOVA

In **MANOVA (Multivariate Analysis of Variance)**, there are two or more dependent variables. For instance, the pain study could include not only the scoring of the relief of pain, but the change in blood pressure.

ANCOVA (Analysis of covariance) "controls for" (removes) the influence of a variable (called the **covariate**) that is correlated with the dependent variable. For example, let's say reaction to pain is correlated with educational level.

To measure the effect of the analgesics, an ANCOVA would determine whether or not the covariate of educational level exerted a significant influence on pain; if so, ANCOVA removes that effect and then determines the significance of the analgesic factor.

There are many variations on these tests, depending on the number of dependent and independent variables, whether the variables are categorical or continuous, and whether a variable that is correlated with the dependent variable needs to be removed (ANCOVA). The bottom line is to look at the p-values to determine if the relationships are statistically significant.

In addition to analyzing the groups as a whole for significance, a variety of tests can do **multiple comparisons**, in which it is possible to determine how any particular group interacts with another, such as comparing the mean of each group with the mean of another group (**Tukey's test**). Other multiple comparison tests include **Dunnett's test**, **Holm's test**, and **Scheffe's test**. Without going into the mathematics, multiple comparison tests, as mentioned, can be presented intuitively in pictorial format, as in **Fig. 15–1**.

CHAPTER 16. CORRELATION AND REGRESSION

Correlation Techniques

Frequently, the researcher asks if there is a correlation between one variable and another, such as weight and blood pressure; or the blood level of homocysteine and the risk for myocardial infarction; or a particular pain level and depression. The data can be ordinal, interval, or ratio.

Correlation coefficient (r) : A **correlation coefficient (r)** is a number between –1 and +1 that describes the degree of correlation between one variable and the other. If there is a perfect positive correlation, as in **Fig. 16–1A**, the correlation coefficient is 1. If there is a perfect negative correlation (**Fig. 16–1B**) the correlation coefficient is –1. If there is no correlation **(Fig. 16–1C**) the correlation is 0.

Commonly, correlation is graphed as a **scattergram**, in which the data points can be visually noted. **Fig. 16–1D**, for instance, shows a positive correlation of 0.85. **Fig. 16–1E** shows a negative correlation of –0.62. A correlation coefficient greater than 0.5 or less than –0.5 is generally considered a strong relationship, while those between 0 and 0.5 or –0.5 are generally considered weak.

Two commonly used types of correlation coefficients are the **Pearson product-moment correlation**, which is used on *interval or ratio data*, and the **Spearman rank-order correlation** (**ρ, rho**), which is used on *ordinal data*. **Mnemonic**: Spearmint (Spearman's) is ordinary (ordinal). The Pearson product-moment correlation is used on linear relationships. If they are not linear, the Pearson correlation will be inaccurate. **Fig. 16–1F**, for instance, shows a nonlinear relationship that is strong but, nevertheless, Pearson would calculate this as a weak relationship using linear correlation techniques. Hence the value in visually inspecting the data. The relations can be linear or non-linear for Spearman's.

The larger the sample size, the closer the correlation coefficient (r) is likely to be to the true population relationship. You can estimate a confidence interval (CI) for the population based on the correlation coefficient of the sample. For instance, if the 95% CI for the correlation coefficient is 0.41 to 0.94, you can be 95% sure that the population correlation coefficient lies within this range. You can also estimate a p-value for the correlation coefficient based on the null hypothesis. Namely, "If the null hypothesis were true and there is no correlation between the variables,

The Correlation Coefficient (r) and Coefficient of Determination (R^2)

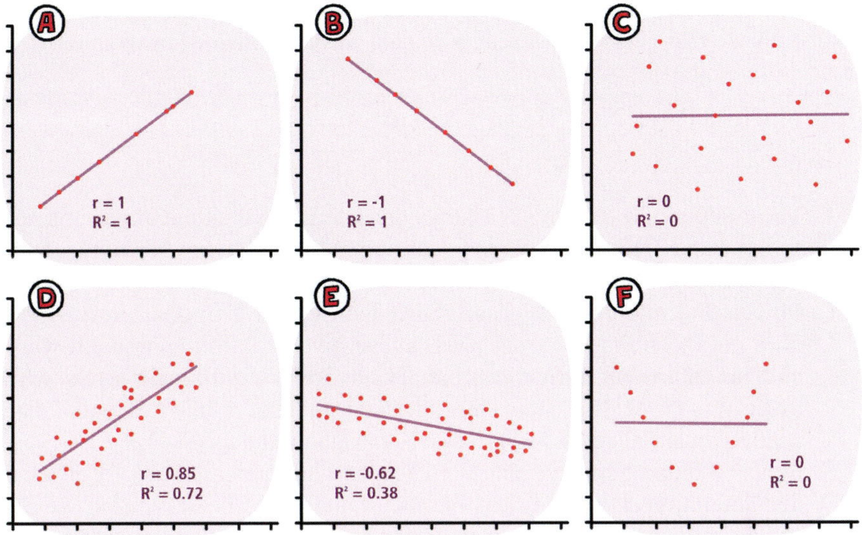

Figure 16–1. The correlation coefficient and coefficient of determination (see text).

what is the chance of obtaining this particular r value for a sample of this size?" If the p-value is low, then reject the null hypothesis and consider that the r that was obtained for the sample is statistically significant.

Coefficient of determination: If a correlation lies somewhere between 0 and 1 (or between 0 and –1), you would like to know why the correlation is not perfect. Some of the imperfect correlation may be due to measurement error or other random factors. The **coefficient of determination** (**r^2**, sometimes written **R^2**), tells you what fraction of the variation of one variable is explained by its relationship to the other variable, as opposed to natural variation within each variable. For instance, if the correlation coefficient (r) between insulin levels and blood sugar is 0.74, then r^2 is $0.74 \times 0.74 = 0.55$. This tells you that 55% of the variability in blood glucose levels is associated with changes in insulin levels, whereas 45% of the variability in blood glucose levels is associated with other factors such as measurement error or natural variability in the concentration of glucose. **R^2** always lies between 0 and 1, since R^2 is a number squared, and r always lies between –1 and +1. A low r^2 value does not necessarily mean the relationship is low; it may just not be linear (**Fig. 16–1F**).

With large samples, a p-value may be less than 0.05 but the effect size may be inconsequential. A tip-off that this is so is a very low r and r^2.

In ANOVA there is a measure of effect size termed **eta-squared (η^2)** , which is analogous to r^2. In the example that compares morphine, hydromorphone, and placebo in pain relief, eta-squared measures the effect of medication as the percentage of variance in the data that we can attribute to a factor, in this case, to medication, as opposed to random variation. While the F-ratio in ANOVA also shows us whether the associations are significant, eta-squared give us more information about how strong that relationship is. Eta-squared is a percentage. Thus, an eta-squared of 37% would indicate that 37% of the variance in pain was explained by medication.

Correlation Does Not Mean Causation

Examples:

1. The number of drownings is highly correlated with the time of year, namely summertime. This does not mean that summertime causes drownings. There are more drownings because more people swim in the summer.
2. Myocardial infarctions are correlated with elevated troponin levels. This does not mean that troponin levels cause myocardial infarctions. It would be a mistake to try to treat heart attacks by lowering troponin levels, when in fact it is the MI that causes the elevated troponins, which leak out of damaged myocardial cells. Too obvious? How about the following:
3. Elevated blood homocysteine is correlated with increased risk for myocardial infarction. Does elevated homocysteine cause heart attacks? Studies designed to decrease homocysteine have not demonstrated any lessening of the risk for MIs. Perhaps a third factor causes a rise in homocysteine as well as a susceptibility to MIs.
4. Elevated LDL cholesterol is correlated with increased risk of cardiovascular disease. But which causes which? If cardiovascular disease causes elevated LDL, or a third factor causes both elevated LDL and cardiovascular disease, then it would not help to try to control arteriosclerosis by taking years of anticholesterol medication. Current medical opinion leans toward LDL cholesterol as a causative act in cardiovascular disease, but there are those who disagree (Kendrick, '07).
5. According to a 2005 study in Finland, women who have abortions are more likely to commit suicide. Do abortions cause suicide, or are women who have abortions more likely to be in social situations that in themselves are more likely to promote suicide? Women who have abortions also are more likely to be murdered and die in accidents. If they are already high-risk for murder, suicide, and accidents, they may be more likely to be in situations where they need an abortion.
6. People often are quick to judge patterns and often attribute causal importance to patterns that are only coincidental. S.G. had an elderly patient who was sure he knew what caused Parkinson's disease; he had purchased his home from someone who had Parkinson's disease, and a year later he, too, was diagnosed with Parkinson's disease. In his mind, it must have been communicable. However, about 1 million people in the USA have Parkinsonism, mostly people over 60. The chance that the person purchased the home from someone with Parkinson's and also would acquire the disease is not so unreasonable, given the number of people who buy homes and the prevalence of Parkinson's disease. In addition, there are thousands of other diseases that both buyer and seller might have had coincidentally. The chance

that at least one of those diseases could have occurred in both buyer and seller is high. The clincher here was pointing out that the spouses of patients with Parkinson's disease do not have a higher incidence of the disease than those not married to someone with Parkinson's. One of the biggest mistakes in research is to confuse correlation with causation.

7. A study indicated that smiling a lot is correlated with a longer life. Should we then go around forcefully smiling at everyone like the Burger King king? Maybe good health induces people to smile more.
8. If people who take DynamoMaxiForte vitamins have a lower risk of illness, is it because of the vitamins or because they take care of their health needs in other ways, such as exercise and a balanced diet?
9. Teenagers who spend a lot of time texting and on social network websites have a higher incidence of sex, stress, substance abuse, depression, and fighting. Should texting be decreased? Which variable causes which?

Criteria of Causality

The epidemiologist Bradford Hill ('65) suggested nine criteria that help establish causality:

1. **Strength of association**. There is a strong association between cause and effect. Hill's example was the increase in scrotal cancer in chimney sweeps.
2. **Temporality**. The effect always follows the cause.
3. **Biologic gradient**. The more intense the exposure to the cause, the greater the effect.
4. **Biologic plausibility**. It helps if the relationship is biologically plausible (but sometimes scientific knowledge at the time may not yet have discovered a plausible mechanism).
5. **Consistency with other knowledge**. Other studies should have repeatedly shown the same relationship.
6. **Biologic coherence**. The proposal of causation should not conflict with known facts about the biology of the disease and how the disease progresses.
7. **Specificity**. Are there other factors that could have caused the disease?
8. **Experimental evidence**. Removal of the harmful substance improves, and addition worsens.
9. **Analogy**. Rubella and thalidomide have been shown to adversely affect early pregnancy. With this analogy, it is easier to consider that other organisms and drugs might do the same.

Question: What kind of test would we use if we wanted to know how blood pressure differs in men and women?

Answer: independent t-test

Question: What kind of test would we use if we wanted to know how blood pressure differs in men and women in three different ethnicities?

Answer: a 2 × 3 between groups ANOVA

Question: What kind of test would we use if we wanted to know how blood pressure differs in diabetic women at dawn, noon, dinnertime, and midnight across the course of the day?

Answer: 1 × 4 within measures (repeated measures) ANOVA

Question: What kind of test would we use if we wanted to measure the correspondence between blood sugar levels and appetite?

Answer: correlation

Regression

Simple linear regression is a method that fits the best straight line through a scattergram collection of data points that are correlated in a linear way; it uses one variable to quantitatively predict the other variable. **Fig. 6–10** is a hypothetical graph that plots the rise in systolic blood pressure with age. The formula for a straight line is:

$$Y = a + bX$$

where *X* is the independent variable (age), *Y* is the dependent variable (blood pressure), *b* (the *regression coefficient*) is the slope of the line, and *a* (the *intercept constant*) is the Y intercept. The equation can be used in this case to calculate the value of the blood pressure that correlates with a given age. Linear regression assumes the relationships are linear. It pays to confirm this visually with a graph.

Two things suggest a relationship between two variables in regression analysis:

1. The slope of the line is not horizontal.
2. The points fall close to the line.

When regression is used on a sample, rather than a population, the question arises as to how well the "best-fit" line on the sample will represent the population. It is possible to calculate a 95% confidence interval for the slope range. For example, if the slope for the sample is 39, a 95% CI might be something like a slope of 18 to 60. Since that range does not include 0, this provides assurance that the correlation is real and not just the result of chance. The larger the sample, the narrower the CI.

An r^2 calculation of, say, 0.56 would tell us that 56% of the correlation can be accounted for by a real linear relationship among the data, while 44% would be due to other factors, such as measurement error, natural variation within the data, or a true relationship that is not linear.

A p-value may also be calculated. To understand what it means, first set up the null hypothesis:

Null hypothesis (H_0): There is no linear correlation between X and Y, and the true slope of the line is 0.

Alternative hypothesis (H_1): There *is* a linear correlation between X and Y, and the true slope of the line is not 0.

Then ask: If the null hypothesis is true, what is the chance of finding a slope this much or further from 0? A $p \leq 0.05$ suggests that the slope most likely is real, and there *is* a linear correlation between X and Y; then reject the null hypothesis.

Correlation and regression techniques are both used to tell if a correlation is significant. Correlation quantifies how variables are related, but does not produce a best-fit line, as does regression. Calculate a linear regression when you want to "weigh" the effect(s) of one (or more) variable(s) on another variable to predict the latter variable.

It is important not to extend the line of best fit beyond the data points. The curve may not be linear beyond those points. In the words of Mark Twain:

> *"In the space of 126 years the Lower Mississippi has shortened itself 242 miles. That is an average of a trifle over one mile and a third per year. Therefore, any calm person, who is not blind or idiotic, can see that in the Old Oolitic Silurian Period, just a million years ago next November, the Lower Mississippi River was upward of 1,300,000 miles long ... and that 742 years from now the Lower Mississippi will be only a mile and three-quarters long..."*

Kinds of Regression Analysis

There are a number of kinds of regression analysis that will not be presented in detail in this book:

Simple nonlinear regression is used on data that are not linear.

In **multiple linear regression**, more than one independent variable is use to predict Y. For instance, blood pressure may depend on the drug dose, age, and other independent variables, all of which are incorporated into the equation:

$Y' = a + bX_1 + bX_2 + bX_3 + bX_4$........etc. depending on the number of variables that affect Y

Multiple nonlinear regression is used to determine correlations among data that are not linear and where there are more than one independent (X) variable.

Logistic regression is used to predict the likelihood of an event in situations where there are two possible ("yes/no-type") results from the influence of multiple independent variables that are tested. The independent variables can be categorical or a mixture of categorical and numeric. For instance, the study may wish to predict the likelihood of stroke ("yes or no"), based on the independent variables of sex, age, and weight (**Fig. 16–2**). The mathematics, which are complex, involve logarithms and the results appear as an odds ratio, and won't be presented here. Most simply, if the odds ratio is higher than 1.0, the independent variable is having an effect on the dependent variable (e.g. age affects the likelihood of stroke). If the odds ratio is less than 1.0, then an increase in the independent variable has a decreased likelihood of the effect. A 95% CI gives the range in which the odds ratio would lie 95% of the time.

Variable #	Question	Units	Odds Ratio	95% CI
1	Sex	0 = female; 1 = male	0.75	0.45 to 0.90
2	Age	0 = <60; 1 = >60	2.10	1.93 to 2.51
3	Weight	lbs	1.65	1.52 to 1.87

Figure 16–2. Logistic regression data (see text).

Regression to the Mean

Fig. 16–3 illustrates the logic trap called **regression to the mean**. It shows how a placebo that has no significant effect on pressure may be made to appear graphically as if it did. **Fig. 16–3A** shows plots of blood pressure of patients who started with different blood pressures, before and after receiving a placebo. There was no significant effect of placebo on the group as a whole. However, **Fig. 16–3B** separates the patients with the lowest initial pressures from the rest of the group and plots their BP before and after receiving the placebo. **Fig. 16–3C** plots the before and after BPs of the patients who had the highest initial BP. It appears that pressures decreased in those with the higher pressures and increased in those with the lowest pressures. The difference is not due to the placebo, but to the fact that blood pressure normally varies from time to time. If the placebo is given when the pressures are low, the pressures will appear higher on average at a later time. If the placebo is given when the pressures are high, the pressures will appear lower on average at a later time, simply because of natural fluctuation, not because of treatment.

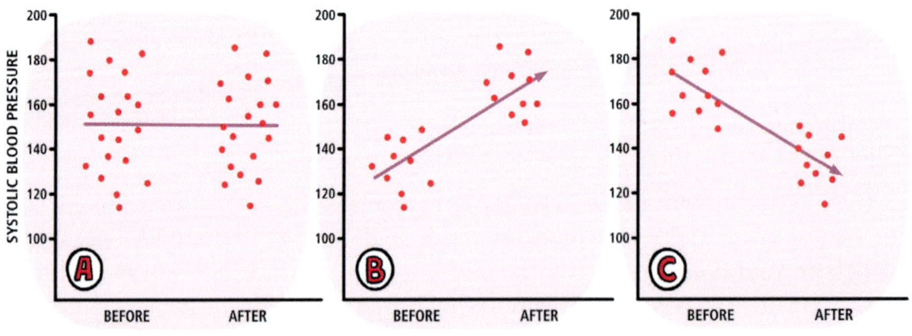

Figure 16–3. Regression to the mean.

CHAPTER 17. NONPARAMETRIC TESTS

T-tests, ANOVA and regression all assume that:

a. the samples are randomly selected
b. the observations are independent (e.g. not people from the same family)
c. the standard deviations of the populations are the same
d. the observations have a reasonably Gaussian (normal) distribution, or at least data that is not too far off from Gaussian. Sometimes you can convert data that is exponential or skewed by plotting the logarithm or square root of the data. But what if you can't do that, and the data clearly are not Gaussian, or you're not sure? You can then use other kinds of tests, termed **nonparametric** tests.

Chi-Square (X^2) Goodness-of-Fit Test

The **chi-square** (X^2) test is used to see if there is a significant association between *categorical* variables, as opposed to continuous variables. Proportions, rather than means, are used to analyze chi-square data. The chi-square **goodness-of-fit** test determines whether the proportions between data categories are significantly different from what would be expected *by theory*.

For instance, as a simple classic example in Mendelian genetics, a new species of medicinal plant is discovered. Two of the plants are crossed. They yield a population of 800 plants, 580 with red seeds and 220 with blue seeds. The categorical variable is seed color, which contains two *levels*, red and blue. We want to test the hypothesis that red genes are dominant and both parent plants are heterozygous for red and blue genes. For example, in the table (**Fig. 17–1**), if the hypothesis is true, one would expect a 3:1 ratio of red to blue seeds, with 600 red seeds and 200 blue seeds. Our null hypothesis is that there is no significant difference between the theorized and observed numbers. The formula is:

X^2 = sum of [(Observed – Expected)^2/Expected]

Thus, $X^2 = (580 - 600)^2/600 + (220 - 200)^2/200 = (-20)^2/600 + (20)^2/200 = .67 + .67 = 1.34$

	Expected	Observed
Red Seeds	600	580
Blue Seeds	200	220

Figure 17–1. Chi-square table (see text).

The computer program will provide a p-value for the resulting 1.34 chi-square number. In this case, p is > 0.05, suggesting that there is no significant statistical difference between your expected seed numbers and the observations. You accept the null hypothesis, and you have acquired evidence for your hypothesis that red seeds are dominant over blue.

The critical X^2 to which you compare the X^2 you calculate can also be looked up in a X^2 table (**Appendix C**) in the appropriate degrees of freedom row. There are 2 categories (rows) in the experiment (red and blue), so df = (n – 1) = 2 – 1 = 1. This corresponds in the X^2 table to a p between 0.10 (10%) and 0.50 (50%) for the calculated X^2 of 1.34. Assuming that you consider an alpha of 0.05 (5%) as the dividing line between significant and nonsignificant, the results indicate that there is no significant statistical difference between your proposed theorized seed numbers and the observations, since the X^2 calculation is less than the table value. You accept the null hypothesis, and you have evidence for your hypothesis that red seeds are dominant over blue.

As another example, say a hospital is studying whether the number of adverse incidents during a 5-year period by the intern staff differs according to the night shift hour. **Fig. 17–2** tabulates the data from 12 midnight to 8 AM (each shift hour is a *level* of the *category* of hours), showing the number of incidents. This is compared with the expected number of incidents, assuming the null hypothesis that there should be no difference that correlates with the hour of night. A chi-square goodness-of-fit test could be used to assess whether or not the observed number of incidents statistically differs significantly from the theorized expected frequency according to the null hypothesis.

Because there are eight levels of the variable shift hours, there are seven degrees of freedom. For an alpha of p = 0.05, the critical X^2 value is 14.07. Our calculated value, $X^2 = 4.57$, is smaller than 14.07. We retain the null and conclude that shift hours are not associated with the number of adverse incidents.

Chi-Square Test of Independence: The **chi-square test of independence** is used to analyze **contingency tables**. A **contingency table** (also called a **crosstabs**

HOURS	# OF INCIDENTS	EXPECTED #
12–1AM	18	21
1AM–2AM	16	21
2AM–3AM	17	21
3AM–4AM	22	21
4AM–5AM	25	21
5AM–6AM	23	21
6AM–7AM	21	21
7AM–8AM	26	21
TOTAL	168	168

Figure 17–2. Ranking in a nonparametric test.

table) is a table displaying two or more categorical variables, which can have an independent/dependent variable relationship:

For instance, the independent variable could be *exposure* (e.g. numbers exposed or not exposed to the risk factor) and the dependent variable *infection* (number becoming infected vs. number not becoming infected).

Or the independent variable might be *treatment* (number of people treated vs. number not treated) and the dependent variable being *cure* (number cured vs. not cured).

As an example, in **Fig. 17–3**, the incidence of breast cancer is compared between the categorical group of *age* (which contains two *levels*, women who had their first child after age 25 and women who had their first child before age 25) and the categorical group of *breast cancer* (which contains two *levels*, breast cancer present or breast cancer absent). The question is whether the incidence of breast cancer is *contingent* upon the age of having the first child. There are two possible outcomes (dependent variables), breast cancer or no breast cancer. Unlike the chi-square goodness-of-fit test, which compares the results against a theoretical expected result, the chi-square test of independence determines whether there is a statistically significant association between two or more categorical variables, in this case age and cancer. The formula resembles the goodness-of-fit test except that the expected values are calculated from the data (not obtained from theory). The chi-square result is again compared with a chi-square table (or a computer program is used) to arrive at a p-value.

X^2 *tests* can be used for tables with more than 2 rows or columns. For instance, in testing 3 new anti-psoriasis drugs, 2 rows might indicate "Number Improved" vs.

Age at First Child	Breast Cancer	No Breast Cancer	TOTAL
25 years +	24	1492	1516
<25 years	58	3478	3536
TOTAL	82	4970	5052

Figure 17–3. Contingency chart for breast cancer (see text).

"Number Not Improved," while 3 columns would represent the number of patients receiving each of the 3 drugs. The degrees of freedom in a contingency table are calculated as the product of (the number of rows – 1) times (the number of columns – 1). In the psoriasis study the df would be (2 – 1) × (3 – 1) = 2.

The chi-square test is not reliable if there are fewer than 5 numbers in any table cell. The numbers should be whole positive numbers and not percentages. The higher the X^2, the lower the p-value. Statisticians disagree about whether the chi-square test should only be used on two-tailed hypotheses or can be used with both two- and one-tailed hypotheses.

A variant of chi-square, called **Fisher's Exact Test**, can be used in a 2 × 2 design (e.g. young women/older women and breast cancer/no breast cancer) when sample size is small (less than 5 or so in any table cell). A **binomial test** is used when there is only one category with two levels, the classic example being the number of heads versus tails in a coin flip. The **McNemar Test** is used when (like the paired t-test) comparisons are done on the same sample, or the two samples are closely matched.

Nonparametric Tests That Use Ranking

The **Mann-Whitney U Test** for comparing two unpaired groups is used when samples from two groups do not have a Gaussian distribution, but you want to know whether or not there is a significant difference between the groups. The Mann-Whitney U test is the nonparametric counterpart to the *unpaired* t-test. Rather than doing calculations with the distribution of data points, the Mann-Whitney test does the calculations on the *ranks* of the numbers, as in **Fig. 17–4.**

In **Fig. 17–4**, the question is whether or not there is a significant difference between samples in group A versus the samples in group B. Since the distributions do not appear to be Gaussian, rather than doing parametric statistics, the numbers are *ranked* and then separated back into groups A and B, summed, and the two columns are compared. The Mann-Whitney U test arrives at a p-value that indicates

RAW DATA		RANKED DATA	
Sample A	**Sample B**	**Sample A**	**Sample B**
4.8	38.4	1.0	7.0
14.6	43.8	2.0	9.5
20.2	43.8	3.0	9.5
28.3	53.7	4.0	13.0
28.5	59.3	5.0	14.0
35.5	60.5	6.0	15.0
39.1	60.6	8.0	16.0
51.9	65.1	11.0	17.0
53.1		12.0	

Figure 17–4. Comparison of raw data with ranked data (see text).

whether or not the groups differ significantly from each another. With a $p \le 0.05$, you conclude that it is unlikely that the groups differ by chance alone.

The **Wilcoxon Test** is the nonparametric counterpart to the *paired* t-test and uses matched ranked pairs. It provides a p-value that indicates whether the difference between the two groups is significant.

The **Spearman Rank Correlation** gives a measure of the correlation between two groups, regardless of whether their relationship is linear or curvilinear **(Pearson's correlation** only measures a linear correlation). Spearman is based on rank and does not assume a Gaussian distribution.

The **Kruskal-Wallis test** is a nonparametric one-way ANOVA test that uses ranking.

Nonparametric tests are less powerful than parametric tests since they use ranking rather than distribution of data points and thereby throw out some of the information. Nonparametric tests should be used when the data are not normal (Gaussian), but it is not always easy to determine normality. The sample size may be too small to tell. Or, the data could seemingly appear non-Gaussian but could be converted to a normal curve (**Fig. 2–3**).

Also, there may be outliers that throw off the normality of the curve, in which case it may pay to analyze the data parametrically without the outliers. A curve does not have to be perfectly Gaussian to use a parametric test, particularly if the sample size is large. Actually, when sample size is large (at least 30 data points in each group), either parametric or nonparametric tests can be used. With smaller sample sizes, parametric tests should be used for Gaussian distributions, while nonparametric tests should be used for non-Gaussian distributions, but the smaller the sample size, the less powerful both tests are. Statisticians sometimes disagree on whether to use a parametric or a nonparametric test.

Nonparametric Tests That Do Not Use Ranking

There are other nonparametric tests that do not use ranking and do not assume a Gaussian distribution (**bootstrapping tests**, **randomization tests**, and **permutation tests**). They are complex computer-run tests that are beyond the scope of this book.

CHAPTER 18. EPIDEMIOLOGICAL TESTS

Epidemiology is the branch of medicine that studies the causes, frequency, distribution, risks, and control of disease in populations. It has its own set of biostatistical terminology.

Incidence vs. Prevalence

Incidence is the *number of new cases* found during a particular *interval of time* (commonly one year) divided by the number of people in the population at risk.

For example, consider a town of 10,000 previously healthy people, where, in 2009, 50 people were affected by a new strain of swine flu, and the flu lasted only about a week:

- The incidence of swine flu in 2009 is 50/10,000 = 0.005 (0.5%). Incidence is a percentage.

Prevalence is the number of cases, new or old, found at a particular *moment* divided by the number of people in the population at risk.

For instance, in the above town:

- The number of people who had swine flu in that town on June 1 of 2009 might be 4 people. The prevalence rate of swine flu on June 1 would only be 4/10,000 = 0.0004 (0.04%), because many people who contracted swine flu prior to June 1 have already gotten better. Moreover, a number of people will not contract it until later that year.

Incidence and prevalence are not the same. If a **chronic** illness widely strikes a population in 2009, but there are no new cases in 2010, the prevalence of the disease for 2010 may be high, even though no one contracted it in 2010, because the disease is chronic, and people who contracted it in 2009 still have it in 2010. The incidence of the disease in 2010 would be 0 because there were no new cases in 2010.

Conversely, an incidence may be high, while the prevalence is extremely low, when assessing a **short-term** disease. For instance, if an acute, fleeting 24-hr illness spreads widely through a population in both 2009 and 2010, the prevalence of the disease at a particular moment in either 2009 or 2010 may be very low at the moment the survey is taken, because many people have already recovered from the disease, or have yet to contract the disease. The incidence of the disease in 2009 and 2010 would be high, though, since there are many new cases of the disease in those years.

As a result, *prevalence* is more useful in evaluating the presence of *chronic* diseases, while *incidence* is more useful for *short-term* diseases. An increasing prevalence rate does not necessarily indicate that a disease is spreading. It may indicate that the disease is lasting longer.

Incidence tells you the risk of contracting the disease; prevalence tells you how widespread the disease is.

Bias in incidence and prevalence figures occurs when a disease is underreported, e.g. because of the social stigma of the disease, or lack of diligence in record keeping.

Incidence and prevalence can be reported as a percentage of a population, or as a ratio, commonly expressed as "per 1,000" or "per 100,000." Incidence is commonly reported "per year," while prevalence is commonly reported over a shorter time interval, e.g. one month or one day, but can be over one year.

Mortality, Morbidity, and Case Fatality

Mortality is the incidence of death in the population at risk. The "population at risk" could refer to all people, or just a particular subset of the population. For instance, "Mortality in patients who had a myocardial infarction in 2009 was 15%."

Morbidity is the same as mortality except that it is the incidence of a particular illness, rather than death, commonly expressed as a percentage.

When a preceding illness is responsible for the mortality (myocardial infarction in this case), mortality is also termed **case fatality rate**. If the population is one that has been exposed to a potentially toxic setting (like food poisoning) the term **attack rate** may be used rather than case fatality rate. For instance, "The attack rate of food poisoning in people who ate at the Sakanna cafeteria party last week was 40%."

Absolute Risk vs. Relative Risk (RR)

A person may want to know the probability that he will contract a particular disease. **Absolute risk** is similar to incidence. For instance if 1 out of 100 smokers will get lung cancer in a lifetime, the absolute risk (incidence rate) of a smoker getting lung cancer in a lifetime is 1%. This contrasts with **relative risk**:

$$\textbf{Relative risk (risk ratio)} = \frac{\text{incidence in people exposed to the risk factor}}{\text{incidence in people not exposed to the risk factor}}$$

For instance, if the incidence of chronic obstructive pulmonary disease (COPD) among smokers is 5% and the incidence of COPD among nonsmokers is 0.05%, then the relative risk of smokers getting COPD is 0.05/0.005 = 10, indicating that smokers are 10 times as likely as non-smokers to get COPD. Relative risk is calculated as a ratio. The absolute risk of COPD would be 5%.

Odds and Odds Ratio (Relative Odds)

Odds differs from *probability*:

The **probability** that a horse will win a race is the fraction of times that you would expect the horse to win. If you expect the horse to win 3 out of 4 times, the probability of winning is 3/4 = 0.75 (75%) of the time. Probability is a percentage.

The **odds** of that horse winning is the number of times you would expect the horse to win divided by the number of times it is expected to lose. In this case the odds are 3/1 = 3, a number rather than a percentage.

Whether computing the probability or the odds, the horse is 3 times more likely to win than lose. A probability has to lie between 0 and 1 (when expressed as decimals). Odds can be anywhere from 0 to infinity.

A clinical **odds ratio** generally refers to the odds that a person with a disease was exposed in the past to the risk factor divided by the odds that the control group had exposure to the risk factor.

Even though relative risk and odds ratio are both ratios, there is a difference between relative risk and odds ratio, as illustrated in the following example. Say that 4 out of 5 smokers will get a heart attack within a certain time period, while 1 out of 5 nonsmokers will get a heart attack in that time period.

The probability of a smoker getting a heart attack is then 4 out of 5, or 0.80 (80%).

The probability of a nonsmoker getting a heart attack is 1 out of 5, or 0.20 (20%).

The odds of a smoker getting a heart attack is 4:1, or 4 (a number, not a percentage).

The odds of a nonsmoker getting a heart attack is 1:4, or .25.

The *relative risk* of a smoker getting a heart attack is then 0.80/0.20 = 4

The *odds ratio* of a smoker getting a heart attack is 4/0.25 = 16 to 1.

Relative risk ratios are more intuitive than odds ratios. In the above example, the relative risk states that a smoker is 4 times more likely to get a heart attack than a nonsmoker, something that is relatively intuitive to grasp. While the odds of a smoker getting a heart attack is also four times that of a nonsmoker, the odds *ratio* is 16, telling you that the odds of a smoker getting a heart attack is 16 times the odds of a nonsmoker getting a heart attack; the number 16 seems too high, and can be confusing.

So why even use odds ratios? Just use relative risk. The problem is that while relative risk assessment can be used in prospective studies, it can't be used in retrospective studies, because, as mentioned:

$$\textbf{Relative risk} = \frac{\text{incidence of the illness in people } \textit{exposed to the risk}}{\text{incidence of the illness in people } \textit{not exposed to the risk}}$$

In order to do a relative risk assessment, you need to know the incidence of the illness in people exposed to the risk. You can know this in a prospective study but not in a retrospective study.

Therefore, odds ratios are used in retrospective studies. You can describe the odds of someone with the illness having had past exposure to the risk factor, and the odds of someone without the illness having had past exposure to the risk factor, which is what you need for an odds ratio.

In practice, if the disease is relatively rare, which is commonly the case, the odds ratio is close to the relative risk, so the terms can be used interchangeably in those cases.

"Smoking is one of the leading causes of statistics."

— F. Knebel

Absolute Risk Reduction (Attributable Risk) vs. Relative Risk Reduction

Absolute risk reduction and *Attributable risk* are the same in that both are the difference between two incidences. They differ in that absolute risk reduction refers to getting better, while attributable risk refers to getting sicker:

Absolute risk reduction is the incidence of disease progression in people taking the placebo minus the incidence of disease progression in people taking the *treatment*. For instance, if the incidence of a smoker who takes a placebo getting lung cancer is 3% and the incidence in a smoker taking a new treatment is 1%, then the absolute risk reduction of the treatment is 3% – 1% = 2% (0.02).

Attributable risk is the incidence of disease attributed to the *risk factor* minus the incidence of the disease in persons not exposed to the risk factor. For instance, if the incidence of a nonsmoker getting lung cancer is 0.5% and the incidence of a smoker getting lung cancer is 3%, the attributable risk of smoking in people with lung cancer is 3% – 0.5% = 2.5% (.025).

Some of the attributable risk can be attributed to random factors in the sampling. How much? Computer programs can calculate a 95% confidence interval, which indicates what the range of difference would be in 95% of repeated trials. If the 95% range does not include 0 difference, the difference is statistically significant.

Recall that relative risk is the incidence of the illness in people *exposed to the risk* divided by the incidence of the illness in people *not exposed to the risk.* Relative risk is a percentage.

Relative risk reduction = (1 – relative risk)

For instance: If the absolute risk (incidence) of death in a person left untreated for a rare pulmonary disease is 0.02 (2%) and the absolute risk (incidence) of death if the person is treated for the disease is 0.002 (0.2%), then the relative risk of death in treated individuals is 0.002/0.02 = 0.1 (10%). The relative risk reduction is 1 – 0.10 = 0.90 (90%). *Sounds like a great treatment!*

Compare this with absolute risk reduction. As mentioned, the absolute risk (incidence) of death when untreated is 0.02 (2%), and the absolute risk (incidence) of the disease when treated is 0.002 (0.2%). The absolute risk reduction of the treatment of the rare disease is only 0.02 – 0.002 = 0.018 (about 1.8%). *Sounds like the treatment is hardly effective!*

So the relative risk reduction is 90%, while the absolute risk reduction is only 1.8%! The reason for the difference is that relative risk reduction is based on proportions, which do not take into account the rarity of a disease, while absolute risk reduction is based on subtraction of percentages, and can be a very small number with a rare disease. It can be confusing, when it is unclear whether relative risk reduction or absolute risk reduction is presented as a research result.

A drug company that wanted to exaggerate the effects of its treatment of a rare disease might list the *relative risk reduction* (90% reduction) rather than the *absolute risk reduction* (a measly 1.8%). It is important to state not only the relative risk (and relative risk reduction) but the absolute risk (and absolute risk reduction). The more uncommon the disease, the greater the discrepancy between relative risk reduction and absolute risk reduction.

Number Needed to Treat (NNT)

$$\textbf{Number needed to treat} = \frac{1}{\text{absolute risk reduction}}$$

The **number needed to treat (NNT)** tells you how many patients would have to be treated for the disease to be prevented in 1 person. For instance, if the absolute risk reduction is 1.8% (0.018), the number of persons needed to treat to prevent one person from getting the disease is 1/0.018 = 56 persons.

If the absolute risk reduction were smaller, say 0.2% (0.002), the NNT would be 1/0.002 = 500. You would then have to treat 500 people to prevent the disease in one person. If the cost of treating one person is $3,000/yr. then you would need to spend $3,000 x 500 people = $1,500,000 to prevent the disease in one person. You have to decide whether the price of treatment is cost-effective. Hence, NNT is valuable information for cost-effectiveness evaluation. When NNT is large, it implies that the therapy is relatively ineffective or the condition is relatively rare.

Number Needed to Harm (NNH)

Related to NNT is **NNH (Number Needed to Harm)**:

$$\textbf{Number needed to harm} = \frac{1}{\text{attributable risk}}$$

For instance, in prescribing antibiotics for strep throat, one study (Newman, '08) found that the NNT was 40,000; namely 40,000 patients would have to be treated to prevent a single case of rheumatic fever. The NNH was 5,000; namely 1 of 5,000 treated patients would experience a severe allergic reaction to the treatment. Should antibiotics be prescribed so liberally for sore throats? NNT and NNH are important considerations in therapeutic decisions.

In contrast with the high NNT for the use of antibiotics for strep throat, the NNT for antibiotic therapy to eradicate H. pylori gastric ulcers is about 1.1; 10 of 11 people with H. pylori will be cured.

Advertisements for the cholesterol-lowering drug Lipitor indicate that it results in about a one third reduction in heart attacks (Carey, '08; Lenzer et al., '10). Sounds good. However, the NNT shows that 100 men would have to be treated for 5 years to prevent a heart attack or stroke in 2 of them (98 of 100 men would receive no benefit). The NNH is important, too, since all the people being treated would also be subject to the potential side effects of the drug, including serious muscle and liver problems. It is unethical for a drug company to mention the percentage improvement but avoid mentioning the NNT. This policy is particularly devious when the company conversely mentions the NNH without indicating the percentage who are harmed. For instance, the company may point to an NNH of 100 (only 1 out of 100 people taking the drug is harmed) but neglect to mention that this same data means a 50% increase in harmful effects when compared with controls.

While these considerations at first glance may raise the question as to whether or not the cholesterol-lowering drug should be used, there are other considerations:

- The greater the number of risk factors that the patient has, the greater the potential usefulness of the drug and the lower may be the NNT for people in that risk group.
- Since the NNT figure applies to only 5 years on the drug, the NNT may be much lower if the patient is on the drug for a longer time, say 30 years. But so may the NNH. You would like to have a low NNT and a high NNH.
- If only 2 of 100 people would benefit from the drug, it means that 20,000 out of 1 million people would benefit. Is it worthwhile to give a drug to a million people to benefit 20,000 people? This is in a sense akin to purchasing a raffle ticket for a charity. It benefits the charity, even though you have only a small chance of winning.

NNT, NNH, and clinical judgment are together important to properly assess the need for a given drug, particularly a lifelong drug, especially in this day of increasing medical expenses.

Sensitivity vs. Specificity

When a clinical test is completely **sensitive**, it means it will detect the disease of interest if the patient has that disease; all people with the disease will test *positive*. There will be no false negatives.

When a test is completely **specific**, it means that people who do not have the disease will all test *negative*; there will be no false positives.

Ideally, a test should be very sensitive and very specific so that there are no false positives or negatives. Typically, tests are not that perfect, so the degree of sensitivity and specificity can be quantified (**Fig. 18–1**):

$$\textbf{Sensitivity} = \frac{\text{(the number of people who have the disease and test positive)}}{\text{(the number of people who have the disease)}}$$

$$\textbf{Specificity} = \frac{\text{(the number of people who do not have the disease and test negative)}}{\text{(the number of people who don't have the disease)}}$$

Sometimes, to deal with false positives and negatives, 2 tests are used, one very sensitive and the other very specific.

1. If the very sensitive test is negative, the patient doesn't have the disease, so go no further.
2. But if the sensitive test is positive, you might be dealing with a false positive. If it's a false positive, this is followed by a (possibly more expensive) test with high specificity, which, if positive, will confirm that the positive is real.

So why not just do the specific test? The specific test may not be very sensitive, and you might miss the diagnosis (get a false negative) with just the specific test.

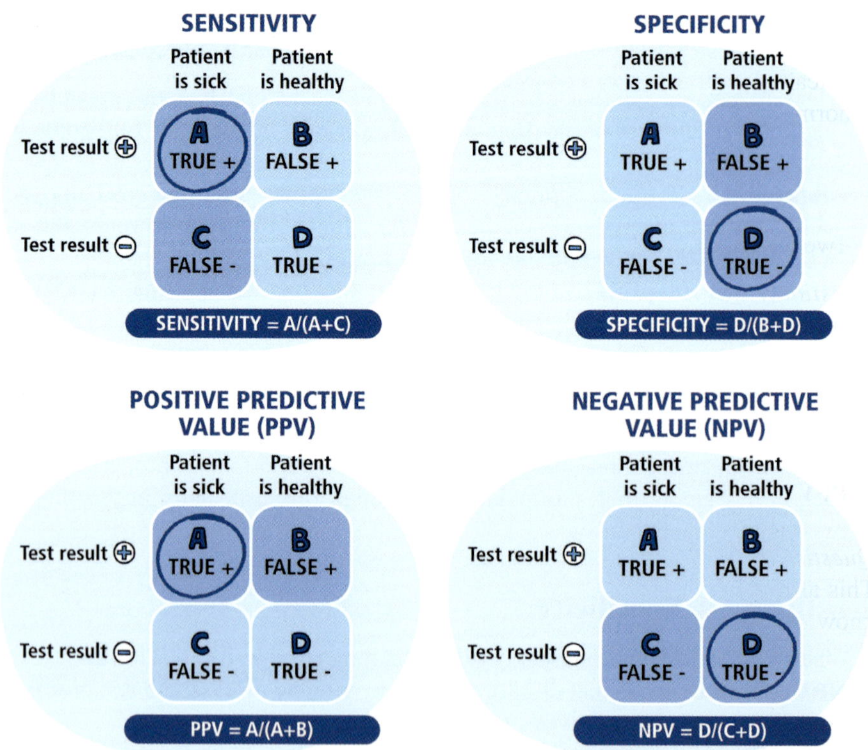

Figure 18–1. Comparison of sensitivity, specificity, positive predictive value, and negative predictive value.

As an example, the ELISA and Western blot-tests are both used in the detection of HIV. ELISA is used initially, since it is relatively sensitive, but there could be a false positive (e.g. in patients with allergies and recent acute illnesses). If positive, ELISA is followed by a more specific confirmatory Western blot-test.

If a test is designed to detect an illness, e.g. diabetes, based on the blood level of glucose, the wider the blood level range that is considered diabetic, the greater the chance of a false positive, i.e. some people without diabetes will fall within the range, and the test will be less specific for diabetes. If the range that is considered diabetic is too narrow, the greater will be the chance of a false negative, i.e. some people with diabetes will be missed; the test will be less sensitive for diabetes. Thus, there is a tradeoff between sensitivity and specificity in the way a test value range is set.

Commonly, laboratory diagnostic tests list a range of normal values, those found in clinically normal people; values outside the range should raise the red flags as to a possible illness. The question is where to draw the line between what is clinically normal and what is not. If the listed normal range is too narrow, some people outside the range will be declared clinically abnormal even if they are not; there will be false positives. If the range of the test is too wide, some people inside the range will be declared clinical normal even if they are not; there will be false negatives.

It is important to remember that someone who falls outside the *statistically* normal range of a particular lab test is not necessarily *clinically* abnormal. The person may just be unusual, but nonetheless clinically normal. It is important for the clinician to not just look at one lab test result, but the constellation of lab tests, physical exam, and history to determine whether or not the patient is clinically abnormal.

Positive and Negative Predictive Values

Two crucial questions:

Question 1: "Doc, I've tested positive for HIV. How likely is it that I have it?" This crucial question is not answered by the specificity or sensitivity of the tests. Unless the test is 100% specific, the specificity of the test doesn't tell you the chance that the patient has HIV. What we want to know is the **positive predictive value** of the test, namely:

$$\mathbf{PPV} = \frac{\text{(number who test positive who have the disease)}}{\text{(number who test positive)}}$$

Question 2: "Doc, I've tested negative for HIV. Does this mean I don't have it?" This also is not answered by the specificity or sensitivity of the test. We want to know the **negative predictive value** of the test, namely:

$$\mathbf{NPV} = \frac{\text{(the number of people who test negative and don't have the disease)}}{\text{(the number of people who test negative)}}$$

The more prevalent the disease is in a population, the higher the positive predictive value and the lower the negative predictive value. The relationships of sensitivity, specificity, PPV and NPV are summarized in **Fig. 18–1**.

PART IV
ARE THE RESEARCH CONCLUSIONS CORRECT?

CHAPTER 19. WHAT'S WRONG HERE?

Darrell Huff ('54) in *How To Lie With Statistics* suggests five general questions to ask in evaluating reports. These also apply to medical reports:

1. Who Says So?
2. How Does the Researcher Know?
3. What's Missing?
4. Did Someone Change The Subject?
5. Does It Make Sense?

1. Who says so?

- Has the researcher received a grant from a pharmaceutical company with a financial interest in the result? Medical conferences and papers commonly require the speaker/writer to reveal what pharmaceutical company affiliations the speaker/author has, to avoid questions of conflict of interest.
- Does the researcher have a financial interest in selling a product related to the research results?
- Is the report from a competing lab, which would get better press by disproving a known positive result rather than duplicating it?
- Are the results published in a reputable, peer-reviewed journal?
- Are previous results correctly quoted? Are they anecdotal? Were they published in reputable peer-reviewed journals?
- Would publishing a statistically nonsignificant result adversely affect the researcher's reputation or career?
- Has the study been confirmed by other labs?

2. How does the researcher know?

- Is there bias in the sampling process? Bias in measurement? Bias in the analysis and interpretation of data?
- Is there adequate sample size (often apparent on a quick look at the data)? While samples may be randomly chosen, the natural variability of the

population may make two small samples markedly different from one another, with different therapeutic results.

- Were survey questions biased? Did people answer honestly? Have only certain people responded to the survey?
- Is the study double-blind?
- Does the study combine data from other experiments that may differ significantly in design from the present one?
- Is the effect big enough to be clinically, not just statistically, significant?
- Does the study just involve men (or just women)? Then it cannot suggest that it applies to women (or men) and children as well.
- Does the paper contain the words "Most studies show...."? This may not be meaningful since journals tend to publish positive results over negative results.
- Does the paper use the vague and unclear phrase "where appropriate"?
- Was the correct statistical test used? Was an unpaired t-test used where a paired t-test was indicated? Were equal sample sizes used for the paired t-test? Were multiple t-tests used where an ANOVA would be more appropriate? Was a chi-square test used when cell counts were less than 5, in which case chi-square is no longer a valid test? Reviewers may not be biostatisticians and may have overlooked an incorrectly applied test. **Fig. 19–1** summarizes the main tests and their indications.
- Has the investigator confused correlation with cause? Heart attacks are correlated with increased blood levels of troponin. But troponin doesn't cause heart attacks; heart attacks cause elevated troponin, which leaks out of damaged cardiac cells. Good handwriting and shoe size are correlated, but one doesn't cause the other. They are both products of growing up and maturing. If there is a correlation between A and B, it doesn't necessarily mean that A causes B. B could cause A, or a third factor C could cause both A and B.
- In the **Hawthorne effect**, patients may strive to perform better when they know they are being observed; the results may not be valid.

3. What's missing?

- Does the paper indicate the sample size?
- Does the paper describe the method of randomization?
- By "randomization" is the researcher referring to random selection from the population, or is the researcher referring to random division into two groups after the random selection from the population is done?
- Were the observations normally distributed (Gaussian)? Independent of one another?
- Were there adequate controls?
- Does the paper define what is meant by "average" (mean, median, or mode)?
- Does the paper report the p-value? A confidence interval?
- Does the paper state whether a one-tailed or a two-tailed t-test was used?

STATISTICAL TESTS	STATISTICAL PROBLEMS
Arithmetic or geometric mean; median; or mode	Calculate an "average"
z-test	Compare one data point or sample mean with the mean of a population of known standard deviation
Single sample t-test	Compare sample mean to a known population mean (Population SD unknown)
Unpaired t-test	Compare means of two distinct samples
Paired t-test	Compare means of two matched samples
Cohen's d; Glass's delta	Calculate effect size
1-way ANOVA	Compare means of more than two groups; one independent variable factor; one dependent variable
2-way ANOVA	Compare means of more than two groups; two independent variable factors; one dependent variable
MANOVA	Compare means of more than two groups; two or more dependent variables
ANCOVA	Control of influence of a covariate in ANOVA test
Pearson product-moment correlation	Correlation between one variable and another; interval or ratio data
Spearman rank-order correlation	Correlation between on variable and another; ordinal data
Simple linear regression	Fit best straight line through a scattergram of linear data
Simple nonlinear regression	Fit best straight line through a scattergram of nonlinear data
Chi-square Goodness of Fit Test	Test association between categorical variables by comparing proportions against proportions predicted by theory
Chi-square Test of Independence	Analyze contingency tables of categorical variables for statistical significance
Fisher's Exact Test	Analyze 2×2 contingency table when cell sample size is less than 5
Binomial Test	Analyze contingency table with 1 category with two levels
McNemar Test	Analyze contingency table with closely matched samples
Mann-Whitney U Test	Compare two *unpaired* groups, when their data do not have a Gaussian distribution
Wilcoxon Test	Compare two *paired* groups, when their data do not have a Gaussian distribution
Kruskal-Wallis Test	ANOVA test that uses ranking
Bootstrapping; randomization tests, permutation tests	Non-parametric tests that do not use ranking

Figure 19–1. Statistical tests and their indications.

- Did the researcher switch from a two-tailed test to a one-tailed test after the experiment was completed without telling anyone, so that the results would appear significant?
- Is the power stated?
- Is an effect size given?
- Did the researcher keep searching, after the project was completed, for a statistical test that would provide his preconceived desired $p < 0.05$?
- How many hypotheses did the researcher look at? Is the study "p-ing all over the place"?
- Were the hypotheses generated *before* the study was completed (the correct way) or *after* (the wrong way)?
- Does the paper mention all the statistical tests that were done on the data?
- Did the researcher add more samples after finding that the results were not significant? Sample size needs to be established prior to the study.
- Does the paper provide raw figures, not just percentages? If 3% of the population got the disease one year and 6% got it the next year, is this a 3% rise or a 100% rise? If 20% of adults smoked in 1980 and 10% smoked in 2000, is this a 10% decrease or a 50% decrease? Just saying "a 50% decrease" is uninterpretable. If a nasal breathing strip is "60% stronger," stronger than what? Than the previous version of the strip? Than a competitor's strip? Than a bandaid? Stronger in adhesion or stronger in spring? Is "60% stronger" compared with something that is already strong or with something that is incredibly weak, thereby making the claim less impressive?
- Has the researcher dismissed negative data, such as trial runs that didn't work, or outliers? You may not know.
- Has survival rate increased because of the treatment or because of earlier detection?
- Pooled data can overlook important information:
  a. "The average person has one ovary and one testicle."
  b. "There has been little progress in finding a cure for cancer." While there may appear to be little progress when lumping all cancers as a whole, there has been considerable progress for certain cancers.
  c. **Simpson's Paradox** (Yule-Simpson, not Homer Simpson): When data from several groups are combined, there may be a paradoxical result. As **Fig. 19–2** shows, drug B was better than drug A in two separate studies. However, when the results of the studies are combined, drug A appears to be better than drug B! This is Simpson's Paradox (d-ohh!), one of the hazards in combining studies.
- Has the paper reported withdrawals from the study?
- Dr. A's surgical operations have a much higher mortality than those of Dr. B. Should we use Dr. B? Not necessarily. Dr. A may by far be the better, more reputable surgeon, which is why the most difficult cases, those with a bad prognosis to begin with, are referred to her. Also, a bad review by only one disgruntled patient may not reflect the views of the majority, who have not volunteered an opinion.

SIMPSON'S PARADOX			
	Study 1% Survival	**Study 2% Survival**	**Combined Studies 1 + 2% Survival**
DRUG A	30/280 = 10.7%	1100/5150 = 21.4%	1130/5330 = 21.2%
DRUG B	95/675 = 14.7%	58/250 = 23.3%	153/925 = 16.5%
Conclusion	B is better drug	B is better drug	A is better drug!

Figure 19–2. Simpson's paradox (see text).

- A report some years ago stated that over 90% of eyeglass prescriptions were incorrect. Incorrect by how much? A clinically nonsignificant amount? Many ophthalmologists purposefully undercorrect high astigmatism, since perfect correction can sometimes be uncomfortable for the patient.
- Are graphics missing baselines? Are graph axes distorted?
- Are there possible causes for the patients' improvement other than the one favored by the author? A decrease in pain could also be due to placebo effect; laying on of the hands; desire of the patient to please the therapist with a favorable report; alternative treatment that the patient was taking at the same time; and spontaneous remissions (most diseases get better by themselves).
- Has the therapist hyped successful cases but said little about bad results (a frequent criticism of research in parapsychology)?
- Does the study just present relative risk (or relative risk reduction), rather than the more meaningful absolute risk (or absolute risk reduction)?
- Does the study state the important statistics of Number Needed to Treat (NNT) and Number Needed to Harm (NNH)?

4. Did someone change the subject?

- If the investigator's subject is the *increase in number of cases*, does the investigator instead provide data for an *increase in reported cases* or *increase in diagnosed cases*, which are not necessarily the same?
- If the subject is improvement in survival with an experimental drug, has the investigator instead provided data for an improvement in a surrogate variable (e.g. reduction in cardiac arrhythmia rather than sudden death)?
- Has *statistical significance* been confused with *clinical significance*?
- Has *statistical abnormality* been confused with *clinical abnormality*?
- If results are statistically nonsignificant, is this confused with "no effect"? A drug may have a significant effect, but it is just not seen because sample size is too small.
- Has a best-fit line been extended beyond the data in regression analysis? If drinking 750 ml of alcohol each day damages the entire brain, it doesn't mean that drinking 30 ml per day damages 4% (30/750) of the brain. If doubling a dosage results in twice the improvement, it doesn't mean that quadrupling the dosage results in quadruple improvement. As mother used to say, "*Too much of anything is no good.*"

5. Does it make sense?

- Drug A is better than drug B with a $p = 0.0529673$. Really? Can one be that accurate about a p-value, or any other biology-related percentage?
- In a report stating that there are 20 million people in the United States with prostate cancer, that would be about 1 case for every male in the 65 and older age group.
- A report indicates that a patient with multiple sclerosis improved temporarily on a new drug. Shall we prescribe the drug, when we know that multiple sclerosis is a disease marked by remissions and exacerbations?
- Is the follow-up long enough? Examples:
  a. In the 1890s a report was published (this is true) of an eye transplant between a rabbit and a human. The published report indicated that 17 days after the surgery the patient "was doing well," to the acclaim of the press. Is this enough time to evaluate such a procedure? Too bad the investigator did not wait another few weeks. (Four other contemporary surgeons jumped on the bandwagon and tried the same procedure.) Enough time has to be given to evaluate a treatment. Many initially approved treatments are discontinued after adverse affects are noted over time.
  b. Surgical and medical approaches to coronary insufficiency are compared, with a 1-year survival follow-up. The medical approach does better. Should we recommend the medical approach? Not necessarily; longer term follow-up may favor the surgical approach, which initially may have adverse peri-operative results.
  c. A cholesterol-lowering drug shows a 1/3 reduction in heart attacks as compared with no treatment, over a 5-year period, with a NNT (Number Needed to Treat) of 50 (50 people would have to be treated to prevent a heart attack in one person). Is 5 years a long enough time to assess the NNT, or for that matter, the NNH (Number Needed to Harm)?
- A drug company studying 100 people reports that 1% of people taking their cholesterol-lowering drug will develop a heart attack in 5 years, while 2% of people not taking the drug will develop a heart attack in 5 years. That is a 50% reduction in heart attacks, based on relative risk, which at a glance sounds great. However, the absolute risk reduction, a more accurate reflection of the efficacy of the drug, is only 1%, since you would have to have 100 people take the drug for 5 years to prevent one heart attack, and there would be side effects and cost of the medication to attend to as well. It is not honest for drug companies to only report relative risk and not absolute risk.
- Infant mortality is less in homes where parents use iPads. Shall parents go out and buy iPads? Homes with iPads are likely to be relatively prosperous and able to afford good medical care.
- A probability cannot be less than 0.

"There are three kinds of lies: lies, damned lies, and statistics."

— B. Disraeli

APPENDIX A. The Z Table

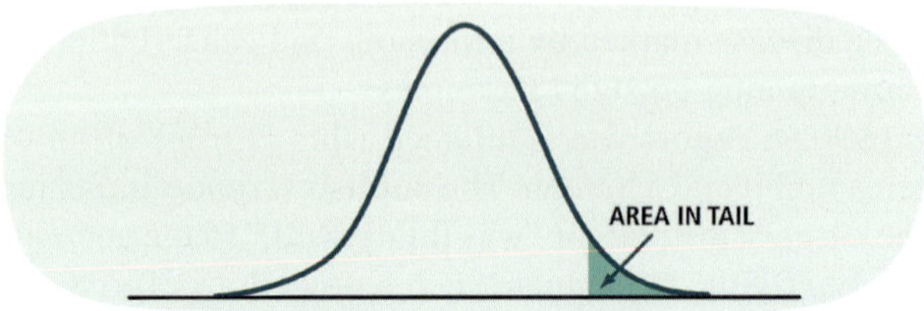

Z Score	Area in Tail	Z Score	Area in Tail
0.00	***.5000 (50%)***	1.55	.0606 (6.06%)
0.05	.4801 (48.01%)	1.60	.0548 (5.48%)
0.10	.4602 (46.02%)	1.65	.0495 (4.95%)
0.15	.4404 (44.04%)	1.70	.0446 (4.46%)
0.20	.4207 (42.07%)	1.75	.0401 (4.01%)
0.25	.4013 (40.13%)	1.80	.0359 (3.59%)
0.30	.3821 (38.21%)	1.85	.0322 (3.22%)
0.35	.3632 (36.32%)	1.90	.0287 (2.87%)
0.40	.3446 (34.46%)	***1.95***	***.0256 (2.56%)***
0.45	.3264 (32.64%)	***2.00***	***.0228 (2.28%)***
0.50	.3085 (30.85%)	2.05	.0202 (2.02%)
0.55	.2912 (29.12%)	2.10	.0179 (1.79%)
0.60	.2743 (27.43%)	2.15	.0158 (1.58%)
0.65	.2578 (25.78%)	2.20	.0139 (1.39%)
0.70	.2420 (24.20%)	2.25	.0122 (1.22%)
0.75	.2266 (22.66%)	2.30	.0107 (1.07%)
0.80	.2119 (21.19%)	2.35	.0094 (0.94%)
0.85	.1977 (19.77%)	2.40	.0082 (0.82%)
0.90	.1841 (18.41%)	2.45	.0071 (0.71%)
0.95	.1711 (17.11%)	2.50	.0062 (0.62%)
1.00	***.1587 (15.87%)***	2.55	.0054 (0.54%)
1.05	.1469 (14.69%)	2.60	.0047 (0.47%)
1.10	.1357 (13.57%)	2.65	.0040 (0.40%)
1.15	.1251 (12.51%)	2.70	.0035 (0.35%)
1.20	.1151 (11.51%)	2.75	.0030 (0.30%)
1.25	.1056 (10.56%)	2.80	.0026 (0.26%)
1.30	.0968 (9.68%)	2.85	.0022 (0.22%)
1.35	.0885 (8.85%)	2.90	.0019 (0.19%)
1.40	.0808 (8.08%)	2.95	.0016 (0.16%)
1.45	.0735 (7.35%)	***3.00***	***.0013 (0.13%)***
1.50	.0668 (6.68%)	3.05	.0011 (0.11%)

APPENDIX B. The t Table

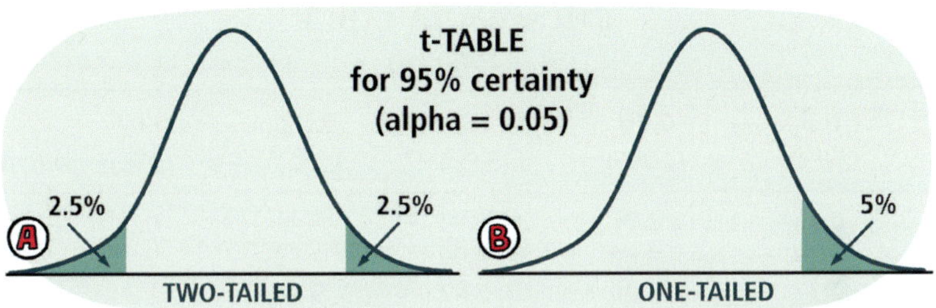

df	Two-Tail Critical t-Value	df	One-Tail Critical t-Value
1	12.706	1	6.314
2	4.303	2	2.920
3	3.182	3	2.353
4	2.776	4	2.132
5	2.571	5	2.015
6	2.447	6	1.943
7	2.365	7	1.895
8	2.306	8	1.860
9	2.262	9	1.833
10	2.228	10	1.812
15	2.131	15	1.753
25	2.060	25	1.708
50	2.009	50	1.676
100	1.984	100	1.660
∞	**1.960**	∞	**1.645**

APPENDIX C. The Chi-Square Table

CHI SQUARE TABLE Alpha (p)						
df	***0.5 (50%)***	***0.10 (10%)***	***0.05 (5%)***	***0.02 (2%)***	***0.01 (1%)***	***0.001 (0.1%)***
1	0.46	2.71	3.84	5.41	6.64	10.83
2	1.39	4.60	5.99	7.82	9.21	13.82
3	2.37	6.25	7.82	9.84	11.34	16.27
4	3.36	7.78	9.49	11.67	13.28	18.47
5	4.35	9.24	11.07	13.39	15.09	20.52
6	5.35	10.64	12.59	15.03	16.81	22.46
7	6.35	12.02	14.07	16.62	18.48	24.32
8	7.34	13.36	15.51	18.17	20.09	26.12
9	8.34	14.68	16.92	19.68	21.67	27.88
10	9.34	15.99	18.31	21.16	23.21	29.59

REFERENCES

Campbell, R. C. (1989) *Statistics for Biologists.* 3rd ed. Cambridge, MA: Cambridge University Press.

Carey, John (2008) *Do Cholesterol Drugs Do Any Good?* http://www.businessweek.com/magazine/content/08_04/b4068052092994.htm

Cohen, J. (1988) *Statistical Power Analysis for the Behavioral Sciences.* 2nd ed. Hillsdale, NJ: Lawrence Erlbaum.

Fisher, R. A. (1949) *The Design of Experiments.* New York: Hafner.

Glaser, Anthony N. (2005) *High-Yield Biostatistics*, Lippincott Williams & Wilkins.

Good, Phillip I. and Hardin, James W. (2009) *Common Errors in Statistics and How to Avoid Them*, Wiley.

Gravetter, F. J. and Wallnau, L. B. (2004) *Statistics for the Behavioral Sciences.* 6th ed. Belmont, CA: Thomson Wadsworth.

Hair, Jr., J. F., Black, W. C., Babin, B. J., Anderson, R. E., and Tatham, R. L. (2006) *Multivariate Data Analysis.* Upper Saddle River, NJ: Pearson Prentice Hall.

Hays, W. L. (1963) *Statistics for the Social Sciences.* 2nd ed. New York: Holt, Rinehart, and Winston.

Hill, Austin Bradford (1965) *The Environment and Disease: Association or Causation?*, Proc Royal Society Medicine 58: 295–300.

Huck, S. W. (2000) *Reading Statistics and Research.* 3rd ed. New York: Addison Wesley Longman.

Huff, Darrell (1954) *How to Lie with Statistics*, W.W. Norton & Co.

Kendrick, Malcolm (2007) The Great Cholesterol Con. John Blake Publishing.

Keppel, G. (1991) *Design and Analysis.* 3rd ed. Englewood Cliffs, NJ: Prentice Hall.

Lang, Thomas A. and Secic, Michelle (2006) *How to Report Statistics in Medicine*, American College of Physicians.

Lenzer, Jeanne and Brownlee, Shannon (2010) *Reckless Medicine*, Discover, Nov: 65–76.

Moore, Thomas J. (1995) *Deadly Medicine*, Simon & Schuster.

Morton, R. F., Hebel, J. R., and Mc Carter, R. J. (1990) *A Study Guide to Epidemiology and Biostatistics.* Gaithersburg, MD: Aspen Publication.

Motulsky, H. (1995) *Intuitive Biostatistics (Ed. 1).* New York: Oxford University Press.

Motulsky, Harvey (2010) *Intuitive Biostatistics (Ed. 2).* New York: Oxford University Press.

Moye, Lemuel A. (2006) *Statistical Reasoning in Medicine: The Intuitive P-Value Primer*, Springer.

Newman, David H. (2008) *Hippocrates' Shadow*; Scribner.

Norman, Geoffrey R. and Streiner, David L. (2008) *Biostatistics: The Bare Essentials*, People's Medical Publishing House.

Pallant, J. (2003) *SPSS Survival Manual*. Maidenhead, PA: Open University Press.

Runyon, R. P., and Haber, A. (1991) *Fundamentals of Behavioral Statistics*. New York: McGraw-Hill.

Siegel, S., and Castellan, Jr., N J. (1988) *Nonparametric Statistics for the Behavioral Sciences*. 2nd ed. New York: McGraw-Hill.

Stevens, J. (1996) *Applied Multivariate Statistics for the Social Sciences*, 3rd ed. Mahway, NJ: Lawrence Erlbaum.

Streiner, David L. and Norman, Geoffrey R. (2003) *PDQ Statistics*, People's Medical Publishing House.

Streiner, David L. and Norman, Geoffrey R. (2009) *PDQ Epidemiology*, People's Medical Publishing House.

Tabachnick, B. G. and Fidell, L. S. (2007) *Using Multivariate Statistics*. 5th ed. Boston, MA: Allyn and Bacon.

Weaver, Ann (2005) *Good-Natured Statistics*, Treasure Island, FL: Jaasas Academic Press.

Weinberg, S. L. and Abramowitz, S. K. (2002*). Data Analysis for the Behavioral Sciences Using SPSS*. Cambridge University Press.

INDEX

RAPID LEARNING AND RETENTION THROUGH THE MEDMASTER SERIES:

BASIC SCIENCES:

CLINICAL NEUROANATOMY MADE RIDICULOUSLY SIMPLE, by S. Goldberg
CLINICAL BIOCHEMISTRY MADE RIDICULOUSLY SIMPLE, by S. Goldberg
ORGANIC CHEMISTRY MADE RIDICULOUSLY SIMPLE, by G.A. Davis
CLINICAL ANATOMY MADE RIDICULOUSLY SIMPLE, by S. Goldberg and H. Ouellette
CLINICAL PHYSIOLOGY MADE RIDICULOUSLY SIMPLE, by S. Goldberg
CLINICAL MICROBIOLOGY MADE RIDICULOUSLY SIMPLE, by M.T. Gladwin, B. Trattler and C.S. Mahan
CLINICAL PHARMACOLOGY MADE RIDICULOUSLY SIMPLE, by J.M. Olson
ACID-BASE, FLUIDS, AND ELECTROLYTES MADE RIDICULOUSLY SIMPLE, by R. Preston
PATHOLOGY MADE RIDICULOUSLY SIMPLE, by A. Zaher
CLINICAL PATHOPHYSIOLOGY MADE RIDICULOUSLY SIMPLE, by A. Berkowitz
CLINICAL BIOSTATISTICS AND EPIDEMIOLOGY MADE RIDICULOUSLY SIMPLE, by A. Weaver and S. Goldberg
HOW CONSCIOUSNESS ARISES: A New Theory of Mind in Humans, Nature, and Machines, by S. Goldberg
CLINICAL GENETICS MADE RIDICULOUSLY SIMPLE, by S. Goldberg
CLINICAL EMBRYOLOGY MADE RIDICULOUSLY SIMPLE, by S. Goldberg

CLINICAL SCIENCES:

OPHTHALMOLOGY MADE RIDICULOUSLY SIMPLE, by S. Goldberg and W. Trattler
PSYCHIATRY MADE RIDICULOUSLY SIMPLE, by J. Nelson, W. Good and M. Ascher
CLINICAL PSYCHOPHARMACOLOGY MADE RIDICULOUSLY SIMPLE, by J. Preston and J. Johnson
BEHAVIORAL MEDICINE MADE RIDICULOUSLY SIMPLE, by F. Seitz and J. Carr
THE FOUR-MINUTE NEUROLOGIC EXAM, by S. Goldberg
CLINICAL RADIOLOGY MADE RIDICULOUSLY SIMPLE, by H. Ouellette and P. Tetreault
THE PRACTITIONER'S POCKET PAL: ULTRA RAPID MEDICAL REFERENCE, by J. Hancock
CLINICAL CARDIOLOGY MADE RIDICULOUSLY SIMPLE, by M.A. Chizner
CARDIAC DRUGS MADE RIDICULOUSLY SIMPLE, by M.A. Chizner and R.E. Chizner
CARDIAC PHYSICAL EXAM MADE RIDICULOUSLY SIMPLE, by M.A. Chizner
ECG INTERPRETATION MADE RIDICULOUSLY SIMPLE, by M.A. Chizner
ORTHOPEDICS MADE RIDICULOUSLY SIMPLE, by P. Tétreault and H. Ouellette
IMMUNOLOGY MADE RIDICULOUSLY SIMPLE, by M. Mahmoudi
ALLERGY AND ASTHMA MADE RIDICULOUSLY SIMPLE, by M. Mahmoudi
RHEUMATOLOGY MADE RIDICULOUSLY SIMPLE, by A.J. Brown
CRITICAL CARE AND HOSPITALIST MEDICINE MADE RIDICULOUSLY SIMPLE, by M. Donahoe and M.T. Gladwin
CLINICAL HEMATOLOGY MADE RIDICULOUSLY SIMPLE, by S. Goldberg
ARE YOU AFRAID OF SNAKES?: A Doctor's Exploration of Alternative Medicine, by C.S. Mahan
WAR AGAINST THE GERMS: EPIDEMICS, MICROORGANISMS, AND BIOWARFARE, by S. Goldberg
ENDOCRINOLOGY MADE RIDICULOUSLY SIMPLE, by S. Goldberg
GASTROENTEROLOGY MADE RIDICULOUSLY SIMPLE, by S. Goldberg
NEUROLOGY MADE RIDICULOUSLY SIMPLE, by S. Goldberg and D. Salzman
ROUTINE LAB VALUES MADE RIDICULOUSLY SIMPLE, by S. Goldberg

BOARD REVIEW:

USMLE STEP 1 MADE RIDICULOUSLY SIMPLE, by A. Carl
USMLE STEP 2 MADE RIDICULOUSLY SIMPLE, by A. Carl
USMLE STEP 3 MADE RIDICULOUSLY SIMPLE, by A. Carl
NCLEX-RN MADE RIDICULOUSLY SIMPLE, by A. Carl

OTHER:

MEDICAL SPANISH MADE RIDICULOUSLY SIMPLE, by T. Espinoza-Abrams
MED SCHOOL MADE RIDICULOUSLY SIMPLE, by S. Goldberg
MED'TOONS (260 humorous medical cartoons by the author) by S. Goldberg
THE STUTTERER'S APPRENTICE, by A. Splaver

For further information, see http://www.medmaster.net or Email: info@medmaster.net.